# Educating for Health

## An Inquiry-Based Approach to PreK-8 Pedagogy

**Valerie A. Ubbes, PhD, CHES**

*Miami University*

Human Kinetics

**Library of Congress Cataloging-in-Publication Data**

Ubbes, Valerie A.
    Educating for health : an inquiry-based approach to preK-8 pedagogy / Valerie A. Ubbes.
        p. cm.
    Includes bibliographical references and index.
    ISBN-13: 978-0-7360-5627-4 (soft cover : alk. paper)
    ISBN-10: 0-7360-5627-0 (soft cover : alk. paper) 1. Health education (Elementary) 2. Health education teachers--Training of. 3. Reflective teaching. I. Title.
    LB1587.A3U33 2008
    372.37'044--dc22

                                              2007047349

ISBN-10: 0-7360-5627-0
ISBN-13: 978-0-7360-5627-4

The Web addresses cited in this text were current as of January 16, 2008, unless otherwise noted.

**Acquisitions Editor:** Bonnie Pettifor Vreeman; **Developmental Editor:** Melissa Feld; **Assistant Editor:** Martha Gullo; **Copyeditor:** Patricia L. MacDonald; **Proofreader:** Erin Cler; **Indexer:** Craig Brown; **Permission Manager:** Dalene Reeder; **Graphic Designer:** Nancy Rasmus; **Graphic Artist:** Dawn Sills; **Cover Designer:** Keith Blomberg; **Photographer (cover):** © Human Kinetics; **Art Manager:** Kelly Hendren; **Associate Art Manager:** Alan L. Wilborn; **Illustrator:** Tammy Page; **Printer:** Versa Press

Printed in the United States of America    10  9  8  7  6  5  4  3  2  1

**Human Kinetics**
Web site: www.HumanKinetics.com

*United States:* Human Kinetics
P.O. Box 5076
Champaign, IL 61825-5076
800-747-4457
e-mail: humank@hkusa.com

*Canada:* Human Kinetics
475 Devonshire Road Unit 100
Windsor, ON N8Y 2L5
800-465-7301 (in Canada only)
e-mail: info@hkcanada.com

*Europe:* Human Kinetics
107 Bradford Road
Stanningley
Leeds LS28 6AT, United Kingdom
+44 (0) 113 255 5665
e-mail: hk@hkeurope.com

*Australia:* Human Kinetics
57A Price Avenue
Lower Mitcham, South Australia 5062
08 8372 0999
e-mail: info@hkaustralia.com

*New Zealand:* Human Kinetics
Division of Sports Distributors NZ Ltd.
P.O. Box 300 226 Albany
North Shore City
Auckland
0064 9 448 1207
e-mail: info@humankinetics.co.nz

In dedication to the Master Teacher:
"I will instruct you and teach you in the way you should go.
I will counsel you with my eye upon you."
*Psalm 32:8*

To RWM, JBP, AM, THE, LJ, and MGF—
with whom I mirrored and anchored
my formative years of identity development;
and to MB—
with whom I articulated the
integrative patterns of wellness
in the choreography of life.

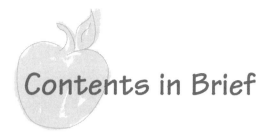

# Contents in Brief

Preface        ix

1   Who We Are: Identity Formation        1

2   Ways to Be: An Ontological Study        21

3   Ways to Think:
    An Epistemological Study        49

4   Ways to Know: Multiple Language
    Forms of Communication        95

5   Ways to Structure Stories:
    Personal and Professional Frameworks    127

6   Ways to Design: Curriculum and
    Pedagogical Frameworks        161

7   Ways to Build Relationships
    Between People and Their Ideas        187

Epilogue        211
References        215
Index        225
About the Author        233

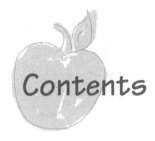

# Contents

Preface    ix

1 **Who We Are: Identity Formation**    1

Teacher as a Changing Learner and Leader 3 • Formation of
Private, Personal, and Public Identities 4 • Goal of Identity Forma-
tion 5 • Epitome of Culture 6 • Conditions That Establish a Quality
of Life 7 • Mystery of Life and Learning 8 • Foster a Culture of
Wellness and Personal Well-Being 9 • Our Sensory-Motor and
Cognitive-Behavioral Responses 10 • Need for Skill Development
When Educating for Health 11 • Change Is Central to Our Lives as
Human Beings 13 • Chapter Features 18

2 **Ways to Be: An Ontological Study**    21

Observing Children as Human Beings 23 • Ways to Be 24 •
Learning Styles 26 • Narratives of Experience 29 • Your Voice Is a
Part of the School's Vision 30 • Human Beings First 30 • Personal
Practical Knowledge 31 • Other Places to Educate for Health 32 •
Ecological Model 32 • Objective Versus Subjective Structures for
Teaching and Learning 35 • Wellness, Well-Being, and Wellness
Space 38 • Hierarchies and Networks Inform Our Work 42 •
Chapter Features 44

3 **Ways to Think:
An Epistemological Study**    49

Constructivist Theory 51 • Constructivism in Education 56 • What
Is Design? 56 • Design as an Inquiry Process 57 • Architectural
Design 58 • Change Orders Are Common 59 • Examples of
Change Orders When Educating for Health 60 • Role of Environ-
ment in Design 62 • Establishing a Learning Environment 63 •

Establish Conditions for Learning 64 • What Is Developmentally Appropriate? 64• What Is Culturally Sensitive? 68 • What Is Body–Brain Compatible? 71 • What Is Health Enhancing? 73 • Thinking as a Health Promoter 74 • Historical Significance of Knowledge Construction 75 • A Story of Professional Integration 78 • Developing a Philosophy to Educate for Health 80 • Design and Style 81 • Role of Literacy in Educating for Health 82 • Objective Knowing and Subjective Knowing 83 • Role of Neuroscience in Constructivist Theory: Zone of Proximal Development 85 • Communication as a Sensory-Motor, Cognitive-Behavioral Approach 86 • Chapter Features 88

## 4 Ways to Know: Multiple Language Forms of Communication 95

Different Signs and Symbols for Language 96 • Structure, Function, and Aesthetic Forms of Language 98 • Intelligence Defined 100 • Domain-Specific Information and Expert Performance 102 • Role of Human Senses in Information Processing 102 • Role of Language and Literacy in Educating for Health 103 • Literacy and Health 104 • Health Communication 106 • A Developmental Perspective of Language as Play 107 • Conceptual Design 108 • Design Problem Solving in Educating for Health 110 • Design for Action Potentials, Action Plans, and Action Research 111 • Habits of Health and Habits of Mind as Possibilities for Healthful Practices 113 • Problems of PreK-12 Health Curriculum 116 • Health Concepts Taught in Other Disciplines 117 • Building an Infrastructure for Health Education 118 • Need for Professional Teaming in Education and Health 119 • Chapter Features 121

## 5 Ways to Structure Stories: Personal and Professional Frameworks 127

Ways to Structure Stories 128 • Use of Children's Literature 129 • Differences Between the Frameworks of Story and Theory 130 • Professional Stories of Health Education 131 • My Professional Philosophy 132 • My Personal Philosophy 133 • Philosophy of How to Educate for Health 134 • Multiple Professional Perspectives in Health 136 • My Interpretation of the Ecological Model 138 • Principles of Practice: The Contextual Model of Human Expertise 141 • Human Beings as Human Doings 144 • Curriculum as Text 145 • Historical and Philosophical Perspectives of Curriculum 147 • Issues of Quality Are a Pattern: Standards and Evidence 149 • Aesthetics Help Build Curriculum Thinking 152 • Chapter Features 158

## 6 Ways to Design: Curriculum and Pedagogical Frameworks 161

Epistemology of Constructivism and Its Relationship to Pedagogy 163 • Pedagogical Content Knowledge 164 • Evidence-Based Instructional Strategies in Health Education 165 • Evidence-Based Instructional Strategies Are Tools and Patterns for All Disciplines 168 • Theoretical Mapping of Three Learning Zones in Educating for Health 172 • Chapter Features 173 • Appendix 176

## 7 Ways to Build Relationships Between People and Their Ideas 187

Relationships With People 191 • Plans for Reflective Practice 193 • Contextual Issues of Space and Place 196 • A River Runs Through You 197 • Relationships Matter 199 • Informed Learning Episodes 202 • Professional Practices That Support a Relational Pedagogy: We Need Each Other 202 • Relationships Take Work 203 • Role of Schools in Building a Safe and Supportive Environment for Learning 205 • Chapter Features 207

Epilogue        211
References      215
Index      225
About the Author      233

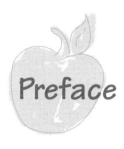

# Preface

The metaphor of a bridge is helpful to this text because the structure of a bridge determines its purpose. Many types of bridges are constructed with many materials. If the purpose (function) is to carry a lot of weight, then the structure of the bridge is reinforced with durable materials. If the purpose is to cross a boundary that cannot be accessed otherwise, then the structure helps to bridge people, places, and things.

In this text, I have purposely crossed bridges to gain access to new information for the profession of health education. As a designer, I looked for how things were made using the language of design. My three-year research process evolved into a transdisciplinary investigation of elements. To communicate my findings to you, I had to find a common language to serve as my schema of major concepts. Those concepts are structure, function, and aesthetics. You will discover how I uncover and use those concepts in several areas of education.

> By staying awake, we keep the larger truths alive. By staying on the journey, we become a living bridge that keeps everything living connected. Not only is our journey essential to us, but each of us is a stitch that keeps the fabric underneath everything whole.
>
> © by Mark Nepo, *The Exquisite Risk: Daring to Live an Authentic Life,* 2005

As an educator, I crossed bridges between education and health to study health education. My work is rich with migratory patterns of bringing ideas from education into health and from health into education. With time and effort, I transformed ideas as the building blocks of knowledge into a theoretical framework for constructing meaning. In uncovering and using educational theories in a health education context, I have been able to look for goodness of fit and to solve problems as I went along. Much of this took place in my classrooms with health and education majors at Miami University. I have also been a voracious reader of books, from picture books to professional books, including journal articles, field trips, and nature as text.

The major problem in education is how to give other people access to what you know, assuming the information is worth knowing. To that end, I have judiciously selected constructivist theory, multiple intelligences theory, and learning styles theory as worthy theoretical frameworks for health education. And I have selected the ecological model of public health as a conceptual framework for migrating theory into education.

As a writer, I have used an inquiry-based approach to investigate the discipline of health education. For the most part, I use personal narrative to explain my scholarly journey. The actual curricular scholarship that evolved into this book is called personal practical knowledge, which has a rich tradition in the work of Connelly and Clandinin (1988). I believe this is one of the most accessible forms of writing for both lay and professional audiences because it leaves little to be translated. This is especially important in my attempt to translate theory from one field to another—education into health and health into education—to form my professional home of health education. This disciplinary language is cumbersome, however, in part because my major premise is that I want professionals outside my discipline to be able to gain access to important foundational knowledge in learning and in life.

To consciously give access to health and education to individuals and groups who may enter the bridge from either side, I have adopted the phrase "educating for health" as an explicit and deliberate attempt to reduce barriers and subtle boundaries that may be perceived in disciplinary jargon. I realize that I also form jargon when I use *educating for health* as a synonym for *health education*, but those readers who are health educators will be stretched to consider the other side more often, which is also my purpose. Admittedly, I am not the first to use the phrase "educating for health." Readers of health education history will recognize the progressive public health work of Matthew Derryberry in the 20th century (Allegrante & Sleet, 2004).

I believe that how we name and frame our discipline of health education is vitally important, and our ability to be flexible and adaptive in all forms of communication makes us progressive. When we structure our standards, our codes of ethics, and our purposes for health education, we form a strong identity for those who wish to join our professional story. However, we must also bring our personal background knowledge into our professional experiences in order to invite a more inclusive and meaningful journey of identity development within the context of community. For example, I bring my personal background knowledge of growing up in a large family and having extensive experience with children, youth, and young adults, informed by age-appropriate developmental theories of Piaget (1954), Vygotsky (1962), and Jung (1923), to advance a preK-8 developmental perspective.

In my early appointment as an assistant professor at Miami University, I tried to integrate my background in physical education, dance, and exercise physiology with health education. I then focused on health education for several years. In my more recent journey as an associate professor, I crossed boundaries from health into education to open up deeper studies in science, math, social studies, and language arts, supported by my childhood experiences in art, music, dance, and sport. This evolving process has enabled me to draw on the richness of knowledge that crosses all eight academic disciplines. For the past 12 years, my Children's Picture Book Database at Miami University (www.lib.muohio.edu/pictbks) has integrated the topics, concepts, and skills of disciplines inclusive to health education. The database, cited as one of the 101 best Web sites for elementary teachers by the International Society for Technology in Education (Lerman, 2005), is based on three major assumptions:

1. The database serves as a technological tool for cognitive construction of meaning by teachers and librarians who need equal access to all disciplines through a meta-language of topics, concepts, and skills for designing curriculum.

2. The database (and the books and Web links it promotes) give learners broader access to subtextual information and communication that promotes a variety of patterned elements (e.g., words, pictures, numbers, body language rhythms, and environmental cues).

3. Some picture books (e.g., narrative text) and informational books (e.g., expository text) offer learners an integrative life experience of human health and wellness in the context of culture, gender, race, ethnicity, and age.

I hope this text bridges your thinking *and* your actions into educating for health. The pedagogical strategies that I model and then explicitly share with you in chapter 6 are one part of the bigger story that you can craft and enjoy in your interactions with young people. I have purposely tried to use multiple forms of information in the design of this book in order to increase its access and utility to an inclusive community of human beings.

Specifically, I hope to accomplish the following goal and objectives with this text: My overall goal is to bridge educational theories into health education, because health educators are indeed educators, by design and by title. Specifically, I introduce professionals who educate for health to intrapersonal and interpersonal theories that will form their cognitive schema for making multiple decisions in pedagogy. I also attempt to change traditional "methods" language to pedagogy so that it is more inclusive of the multiple processes of teaching, especially the way pedagogy is informed by educational theories that I have been mapping into health education. For example, I coauthored the first paper on constructivism in health education (Ubbes, Black, & Ausherman, 1999) and wrote the first book on multiple intelligences in health education (Ubbes, 2004). These theories are developed more fully in this text, along with learning styles and evidence-based instructional strategies.

My other objectives include the following:

• To show how an ecological model from public health and the four conditions for learning establish macro- and microenvironments, respectively, for pedagogical design.

• To establish the preparation of professionals as a personal narrative of practical knowledge that empowers an active voice—participatory and inquiry based.

• To advance the process of educating for health as a transforming journey of many professionals who share concepts, theories, and pedagogies in educational disciplines that study health as a concept—and who could promote health investigations with their learners for enhanced personal and cultural outcomes.

• To promote health education as a synergistic focus on human beings in the curriculum of life *and* as a structured place and time in the school curriculum, where children and youth are the living subjects of study in critical need of health-related skill development (e.g., habits of mind) and health-related content (e.g., habits of health).

• To integrate pedagogy with a philosophy of educating for health so that professionals are encouraged to think through this synthesis work from an inner core of identity formation early and continually in their careers. Without a philosophy of health, one will *not* teach or promote health no matter what! Educators need to learn how to think about health and why it matters to their effectiveness as human beings and as professionals who can advocate for a culture of wellness as foundational to learning.

• To support the growth and development of children through a sensory-motor, cognitive-behavioral approach to human health and well-being, guided by professionals who appreciate the role of neuroscience in learning how to learn (Willis, 2006).

• To use communication, conflict resolution, and stress management skills as a subtext in the book because educators need support in negotiating their professional careers, including how to teach young people to demonstrate health-enhancing skills in a changing world.

- To establish an inquiry-based approach to educating for health as a goal for all human beings, especially educators who have been called to teach a relational pedagogy.

May your journey be rich and rewarding. Please share your own stories with me by e-mail.

Valerie A. Ubbes, PhD, CHES
ubbesva@muohio.edu

# Who We Are:
# Identity Formation

This meeting of our inner and outer lives is called integrity, and the health of our integrity often determines our inner strength and resilience in meeting the outer world. This is the purpose of integrity: to balance the outer forces of existence with the inner forces of spirit.

© by Mark Nepo, *The Exquisite Risk: Daring to Live an Authentic Life*, 2005

Remember what it felt like to walk onto the college campus as a newbie? Perhaps it was a year or two ago, or maybe it was many years ago. What did those first few days of change mean to you? How did the excitement and the fear of the experience imprint in your mind?

You have many stories to tell: the stories of your first roommate's perspectives, your first university class, your first college romance, your first concert or sporting event, your first call home, your first exam. These stories of firsts are among the other changes in your life. Some experiences linger, but you are measured by your next developmental readiness to learn about life. Human beings are on a quest to know and be known, to love and be loved, on their journey into the unknown.

This book is about your personal development as a professional who will educate for health. It is an ambitious endeavor because it assumes you are a professional who knows the next step and the next task to undertake. But it need not be framed from that overwhelming charge. What if you sign up for the expedition with an open mind and an open vulnerability to self-discovery? What if you simply keep track of the changes you experience this semester and reflect a bit on those, weighing the possibility for growth and development? What if you are asked to simply come to know yourself a little more in this journey—to be willing to take yourself into five dimensions of well-being and seek a higher quality of life by looking for evidence of social, emotional, intellectual, physical, and spiritual space in your daily walks and experiences around campus?

This simple but difficult request is your small story in a bigger story of life. That is to say, you are living one day in your life either fully formed as a human being or limited by a narrow scope of who you are. You have a fabulous opportunity to live each day more fully through a wider interpretation of your day. When defined by multiple perspectives of social interactions, physical interactions, intellectual interactions, and so forth, your day can't let you down. Nor should you let yourself down by taking an expedition with a narrow interpretation of life.

Investigations into selfhood begin at birth but are more meaningful when you enter collegiate life. It is here where you form your early adult friendships and try on many ideas as if you were trying on the latest fashions. Some fashions look good on someone else, you reason, but not on you. Yet your friends, both inside and outside the classroom, show you the possibilities for making them work for you too. Even faculty and professionals challenge you to consider the opportunities for the latest and greatest theory, book, or career choice.

If you want to know what tomorrow holds, live today. If you want to know what yesterday meant, live today. There is only the present to negotiate, so keep your life transparent to the kaleidoscope of possibilities. If the light doesn't show through today, it may tomorrow when you have a better background knowledge of the topic, concept, or skill. When your life is transparent, it is capable of transmitting light so that objects on the other side can be seen clearly. If your personal story is transparent, it is so fine in texture that it can be seen through, just as a sheer fabric can be seen through. If you sense that your story lacks clarity, talk with another human being who can be candid and open from his perspective. But don't be limited by one interaction when you can ask others for their thoughts or experiences. Transparency means you can learn to see through to the other side as long as you realize there is another side to the day, the issue, the problem, the cause.

## Teacher as a Changing Learner and Leader

My reason for writing this book is simple: Unless you have the motivation to learn about yourself as a human being, there is little reason for you to become a teacher. A teacher is a learner first and always. A teacher is also a leader who models how to grow and change on a daily basis. Palmer (1998) reminds us, "Good teachers join self and subject and students in the fabric of life" (p. 11).

As a health educator, I have learned that the content of my vocation is based on the contentment of my soul. If I am well, I walk into classrooms with the eagerness to share space and place in an open exchange of teaching and learning. If I am less well on any given day, even to the point of feeling stressed or conflicted by a recent event, then I walk into classrooms with a shadow to cast over my learners. However, if the goal is to be transparent so that the texture of our interactions is seen clearly by all who are present, then I will create a space that invites a mutual sharing of stories, theories, and perspectives to the hour.

Since health and well-being are a personal journey, we must be mindful of our own space and notice how our multiple roles and identities help or hinder these interactions. Palmer illuminates this reality by suggesting the following:

> A good teacher must stand where personal and public meet, dealing with a thundering flow of traffic at an intersection where "weaving a web of connectedness" feels more like crossing a freeway on foot. As we try to connect ourselves and our subjects with our students, we make ourselves, as well as our subjects, vulnerable to indifference, judgment, ridicule. To reduce our vulnerability, we disconnect from students, from subjects, and even ourselves. We build a wall between inner truth and outer performance, and we play-act the teacher's part. (p. 17)

Nepo (2005) suggests how to deal with life changes: "Part of our dance as human beings is to live in full acceptance of the fact that nothing,

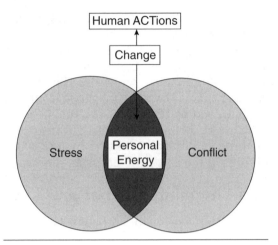

**Figure 1.1**    Relationship between stress and conflict.

not even the earth beneath our feet, is standing still" (p. 84). Figure 1.1 shows how a life change (also known as a metamorphosis) emerges from the personal energy of a human being experiencing normal daily stress or conflict. The effects of the stress or conflict have the capacity to create positive and negative outcomes, both of which can contribute to change. Stress, conflict, and energy are important concepts to know and understand in life because they help to change our human ACTions. In health education, stress management and conflict management skills can be practiced because the curriculum addresses human stress and conflict, as well as communication skills (see page 12).

## Formation of Private, Personal, and Public Identities

The curriculum of life is health. To educate for health, we must help individuals name their private, personal, and public identities (figure 1.2). Private identity is grounded in solitude and silence, meditative reading, walking in the woods or sitting by a lake, keeping a journal, and finding a friend who will listen (Palmer, 1998). These are ways to talk to yourself so you can learn to author the stories within you. Personal identity is your self-identity within your intrapersonal space. In contrast, your public identity is your cultural identity within your interpersonal space. Each of your private, personal, and public identities can interrelate with each other. Most often, your personal and public identities are present in the classroom for engagement with other learners.

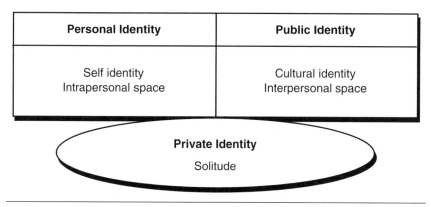

**Figure 1.2** Private, personal, and public identity.

## Goal of Identity Formation

The goal of identity formation is to learn how to author your own story about who you are in a variety of settings and places throughout your day. It is natural to feel more comfortable in some situations than others. As you learn to recognize your own signs, signals, and patterns of stress in your physical, social, intellectual, spiritual, and emotional being, you learn more about yourself. When we develop an internal frame of reference, we are able to increase our sense of self-control in dealing with life's ongoing stressors instead of feeling victimized.

By their very nature, certain things evoke a negative emotional response. Of all the sounds available to our ears to hear, the siren of an ambulance or an emergency response vehicle brings us a moment of concern and maybe even an outward expression of words: "I hope everyone is okay." Some of us may even transform our hope into an act of faith by offering a quiet moment of reflection or prayer. Moments of reflection vary among faiths. The Islamic tradition has a ritual of five pauses in the day during which adherents, standing and facing in the direction of Mecca, show their respect and faith. Muslims follow the weekly convention of Friday congregation. The Hebrew tradition has a practice of using sundown on Fridays to sundown on Saturdays as a natural pattern for gathering in the community. And the Christian tradition with its multiple denominations varies widely in its patterned response to tradition, faith, and hope, usually gathering in community on Sundays and often in midweek.

These different days of the week for faith communities form differently in the educational community. Schools identified as public, private, or parochial are also flanked by traditions of schooling at home. The rhythm of school attendance varies by structure and function: year-round schooling, weekend schooling for extended or remedial learning, and the traditional 10-month cycle of education with 180 days and a variety of vacations and holidays.

When the United States experienced an attack on the Twin Towers of the World Trade Center on September 11, 2001, the world was stunned. Moved to tears and to action, people of all cultural backgrounds, of various ages and abilities, crossed boundaries to reach out with caring concern to those who were most affected by the disaster. Since then, many natural disasters, in the form of tsunamis, earthquakes, and hurricanes, have continued to remind us of the devastation and impact of powerful forces that cannot be explained fully by psychology, sociology, ethics, biology, meteorology, geology, and other disciplinary studies. We must continue to acknowledge the value of a community of experts who share interdisciplinary knowledge (the prefix *inter* meaning between), especially when life cannot be explained by only one perspective. When we expand our interdisciplinary knowledge into opportunities for intercultural, interfaith, and international experiences, we gain an interdependence that is reciprocal and renewing.

We are designed as potential agents of social and historical change. Each day, we can learn to harness our human potential to solve problems and fashion products that are valued in one or more cultures (Gardner, 1993). As human beings, we are who we are, rich in diversity, each of us with differentiated potential to contribute our gifts and talents to the world. In professional development, we must reduce our tendencies to be only "human doings." Who we are is just as important as what we do when working with young people. Our positive role modeling will help our youth mature into responsible citizens in their homes, schools, communities, and countries during their formative years.

## Epitome of Culture

Some of the greatest mysteries of life are unraveled when accomplished scientists, musicians, and artists come together to celebrate a cause (e.g., world hunger) or when whole communities, regardless of their backgrounds, gather in the wake of unexpected events (e.g., hurricanes and tsunamis). These moments of truth seeking, when individuals construct the world by making meaning and solving problems, become the epitome of culture. Formed by our individual knowledge, beliefs, and behaviors, culture depends on our capacity to learn and transmit knowledge to future generations.

After the September 11 disaster in New York City, children and youth in the city's schools were thrust into an environment of chaos and confusion. Teachers, staff, administrators, and health professionals did not have the answers for young people. Both young and old became equals in the challenge to survive, interact, and make sense of the day. The typical structure of schooling as they knew it was leveled. The subsequent co-constructions of growth and renewal were not scripted. Daily decisions were made around who, what, where, when, why, and how. For the adults, life became the curriculum. For the children, returning the ashes and rubble to new forms of life became constructions of deeper meaning and common sense (Harwayne & New York City Board of Education, 2002). As young and old joined hands to survive, the darkness of the dis-*aster* (from Latin, meaning *star*) transformed into enlightened places of living and learning with each successive day.

Each of us—from our own perspectives, places, and positions on the planet—sees the world differently. We are called to a "hidden wholeness," which Merton (1989, p. 506) named and Palmer (1998) refined in the context of education. Palmer begins with the example of breathing as a form of paradox, "requiring inhaling and exhaling to be whole. . . . hold them together, and they generate the energy of life: pull them apart, and the current [energy] stops flowing" (pp. 63, 65). Palmer explains how the world of education is filled with broken paradoxes (e.g., we separate head from heart, facts from feelings, theory from practice, and teaching from learning). He urges us all toward a creative synthesis of paradoxical thinking, which "requires that we embrace a view of the world in which opposites are joined, so that we can see the world clearly and see it whole" (p. 66).

Young children are not adept at seeing and understanding the abstract world—they see only the concrete until their midteens. Returning to the September 11 example, many kids experienced the disturbing visual on television of an airplane crashing into the Twin Towers of the World Trade Center in New York City. Some kids experienced it firsthand in concrete form, and many other children gave eye-witness accounts after seeing and hearing concrete media coverage of the event. Whether an event is unnatural (e.g., September 11) or a natural disaster (e.g., frequent hurricanes in Florida and New Orleans), many children and youth continue to experience stress in intense forms.

## Conditions That Establish a Quality of Life

Stress can be a shadow on the growth and development of young people. Stress is a perceived pressure or system of forces that strains or cripples a human nervous system. Organisms and humans can be resilient when under pressure if the environmental conditions that cause stress are adaptive and supportive. If a human being is already under pressure and an additional force is placed on that person, then her nervous system has to work overtime, along with the immune and endocrine systems, to negotiate the external and internal forces on the body and brain. The human nervous system mediates and works in tandem with nine other body systems to keep the brain and body functioning. A supportive physical environment of adequate lighting, proper temperatures, food, water, and shelter is essential to our lives, but we also need supportive human relationships grounded in love and compassion to help us process and negotiate stress. If excessive pressures of physical stress and human conflict are frequently combined, the resulting consequences can compromise our quality of life and become life threatening.

Stress can be a force of great significance that helps move people to positive action. Palmer's view of a possible life stressor is the tension that results when a positive experience and negative experience are held together in a paradox (from Greek *paradoxos*, conflicting with expectation). Rather than seeing the opposites and focusing on the tensions between them, enlightened learners, both young and old, can learn to join contradictions into a hidden wholeness. The mystery found between, among, and within the opposites can be respected and appreciated—sometimes with faith—and often are made possible through trust in the abstract.

## Mystery of Life and Learning

Here's how humans can enter into this mystery of life and learning. Words are the voice of the heart. Words, of course, are formed in our brains, but our hearts keep the pace and rhythm of life flowing outward into the body so our words and actions can line up. Each of us has been moved by our thoughts. We move because our sensory systems bring the sights, sounds, smells, tastes, and touches to the thalamus and other limbic structures deep in the brain in order to sort the information into supportive or threatening responses. Within milliseconds, the frontal cortex helps us think about what needs to be done with the information coming in, even though so much of the sensory information is sorted and dumped without our attending to it consciously.

Where and how we choose to focus our thoughts and feelings make a big difference in how effective we will be in life. We can learn to think with our supportive or conflicted feelings, but the results are not as powerful as when we learn to think with thoughts *and* feelings. Feelings play a supportive role in our thinking, as suggested by this account: "It is widely assumed that emotion and rationality are somehow opposed to each other, and that rational decisions are better than emotional ones. In fact, emotion and reason work closely together" (*Economist*, 2006, p. 7).

When we teach young people to think holistically about information, we give them time and tools to construct meaning about how *they* think, feel, and act regarding the information. In today's educational culture, we have isolated the emotions from the intellect to such a degree that some teachers, and certainly most of their students, are acting to learn information that has been thought out and delivered to them from somewhere else. Fortunately, many veteran educators and administrators have given young people access to their personal questions and motivations to learn, acknowledging a co-curriculum of reciprocal teaching and learning. To determine the journey for others every day is to violate how each of us can learn to function as dynamic human beings by using the answers within us. Along with this freedom to think and act, we can also learn to exercise self-control and responsibilities for our positive and negative actions.

Learning begins and ends with each individual. We can target the masses with our educational messages, but each sound byte, visual byte, and kinesthetic byte of information must be attended to and organized by and learned by each student. This individual tailoring of the information to be learned cannot be coerced or cajoled into knowing or feeling or acting. The learner, in tandem with her supportive network of caring adults and peers, can make learning a delight, or she can make it pure drudgery. Although knowledge is socially constructed, each learner must choose to take the first step and the subsequent steps on the journey to learning and to life.

## Foster a Culture of Wellness and Personal Well-Being

Perhaps the real balancing act in education is honoring the paradox of self and others. This dualism may be too simplistic in the context of wellness, which honors each human being for his or her multiple beings: physical being, social being, intellectual being, spiritual being, and emotional being. When we educate for health, the emotions and the intellect are joined by the social support of others, a healthy spirit of one's self in the world, and a healthy physical organism. Therefore, in the hidden wholeness of being a human, the spiritual self emerges emotionally, intellectually, and physically to feel, think, and act in the context of the social world. In this text, the dualisms of personal and cultural are used to embrace how each person can seek wellness through his or her multiple beings within a culture. When humans seek personal well-being as a daily life goal, we help foster a culture of wellness in the world.

The way we interpret concepts and practice health-related skills in various cultural contexts determines how well we live our lives. We are shaped by the thoughts, words, and actions of our own brains and supported or not by the thoughts, words, and actions of others. How we negotiate for ourselves in the context of others brings us into maturity as we age and as we grow to understand who we are and who we want to become. In the days, nights, and shadows of life, the decision is ours. Each of us enters the world with a voice and a choice. True, some people have more opportunities for voice and choice, but we are wholesomely alive to choose our own destinies within the design of the universe.

## Our Sensory-Motor and Cognitive-Behavioral Responses

The learning conditions for growth and development are nurtured within a personal and cultural context. That is to say, beginning at infancy, each of us needs personal and cultural interactions that support our potential for life. Information comes "in" to our sensory organs as different forms of potential energy—sights, sounds, smells, tastes, and touches—then transforms into a series of action potentials. Sensory information is translated from waves of light or sound into the actions of seeing and hearing, respectively, with the help of our brains. Such sensory-motor impulses become cognitive-behavioral patterns of thoughts and actions. As long as we are not threatened or overloaded with sensory stimuli, we have the cognitive ability to focus and process our thoughts into health-enhancing behaviors.

Our thought processes can lead to action. We sometimes act on what we see. We sometimes act on what we hear. We sometimes act on what we smell. We sometimes act on what we taste. We sometimes act on what we touch. Whatever we do, we are consciously thinking and choosing to act (unless the action involves a reflex to keep our bodies and brains safe).

Constantly changing environmental information grabs the attention of our brains and bodies (or not) to determine a quality of life that is there for our choosing. We must certainly guide and teach our young people how to respond and process the pleasures and pains of life's experiences. As education and health professionals, we are a supportive network for transforming sound bytes, visual images, and supportive touches into health-enhancing messages for the growth and development of children and youth.

# Need for Skill Development
# When Educating for Health

When we educate for health, we need to promote the health-related skills of decision making, goal setting, communication, conflict resolution, and stress management in explicit ways so students will have practice time to improve their quality of life. Health educators need to have more time to teach these health-related skills in preK-8 classrooms. Parents and health professionals can also team with health educators as role models for guiding young people through the healthy and unhealthy choices of life.

In this next section, you will learn about your change potential through the skill development of communication, stress management, and conflict management. Figure 1.3 shows how the five conflict response styles can be organized by the degree to which we attempt to satisfy our own concerns and the degree to which we attempt to satisfy others' concerns. In our use of these different response styles, we can model uncooperative and cooperative actions and assertive and unassertive actions. Table

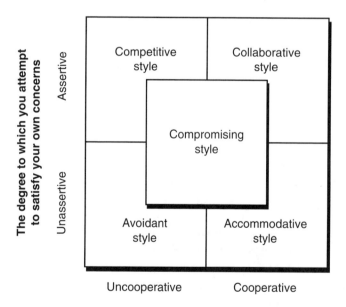

**Figure 1.3**   Conflict response styles: How we respond to conflict. This grid can be used to identify your style or anyone else's.

Reprinted, by permission, from T. Wheeler, 2004, *Conflict response styles grid* (Columbus, OH: Ohio Commission for Dispute Resolution and Conflict Management).

# Communication Skills for Managing Conflict

## NAME, CLAIM, REFRAME, TAME, AIM, AND DON'T BLAME!

Feelings are arguably the hardest thing to manage when in conflict with others. The following process looks at the concepts of communication and relationships; the topics of social, emotional, and intellectual health; and the skills of communication and conflict resolution.

Adolescents can use the rhythm of these words to assess and practice how well they "name, claim, reframe, tame, aim, and (don't) blame!" their feelings:

1. Name the feeling. What, exactly, am I feeling? What's going on here?

2. Claim the feeling. This is my feeling. No one made me feel this way. How I am feeling is my response (e.g., anger, sadness, frustration) to this conflict situation. My feeling may or may not be an appropriate response in this situation, but I acknowledge that it is still mine. (For some who have developed the habit of dealing with feelings cerebrally, there is an additional step of allowing themselves to actually feel the emotion.)

3. Reframe the feeling. Is this the first time I have felt this way? What are the specific factors of this conflict? Is there a history of previous conflicts with this individual that intensifies my present feelings? Can I reframe my present feelings in such a way that they become helpful in resolving the current conflict? Is it appropriate for me to reframe my feelings in this situation?

4. Tame the feeling. If you are uncomfortable with the intensity of your feelings, you can do things to reduce their intensity. Jogging, playing racquetball, swimming, and cleaning are some possible ways to release intense negative energy so that feelings can be reframed and aimed.

5. Aim the feeling. What am I going to do with my feelings? Will I talk this out with someone? Do I need to understand my part in the conflict? Will I ask the other party to work with me to resolve it? Will I decide to do something differently next time? All of these are ways of aiming.

6. Don't blame! Be responsible with your thoughts and feelings, and apologize for your role in the conflict. Forgiveness is a gift you give to others. Forgiving is for *giving*. As you respect and honor another human being in the present, you gain freedom from the past and clear the way for a better future.

Adapted, by permission, from T. Wheeler, 1995, *Name, claim, reframe, tame, aim, don't blame* (Columbus, OH: Ohio Commission for Dispute Resolution and Conflict Management), 54.

Table 1.1   **Passive, Assertive, and Aggressive Actions**

| Passive | Assertive | Aggressive |
|---|---|---|
| To let others choose for you | To advocate and choose for yourself | To choose for another |

1.1 shows you the difference between assertive, passive, and aggressive communication styles. Figure 1.4 shows how you can use the metaphor of animal behaviors to teach young people about five conflict response styles that people use when communicating with others. The goal of each of these conflict resolution tools is to show you how to communicate more effectively in your relationships with others. As you gain experience and success with these skills, you will be able to use them to educate others for health and well-being.

# Change Is Central to Our Lives as Human Beings

Change is an essential part of life that is often despised by human beings under stress or in conflict. But when we educate others for a journey of health, we can give them time to understand that change is central to our lives as human beings. How we honor and negotiate change determines whether we function in healthy ways—leading to a quality of life that advances wellness—or in harmful ways.

The concept of change can be described as a metamorphosis of structure, function, and aesthetics. As shown in figure 1.5, the symbol of a triangle shows these three elements of design. As the elements change, or "morph," the design emerges. *Delta*, the symbol for the fourth letter in the Greek alphabet, is represented by a triangle. *Delta* also refers to the fertile land at the mouth of a river formed by changing deposits of mud, sand, and pebbles. Deltas in rivers are often in the shape of a triangle. As human beings, we need to structure each 24-hour day so that our five dimensions of well-being help us to function in health-enhancing ways, leading to an aesthetic quality of life.

As adults, if we are afraid of change or fail to realize the benefits of change, we will not be effective change agents for children. As professionals who educate for health, we must incrementally reveal the benefits of change to young people. If a change is more than we can cope with at any given time, it will be obvious; words, feelings, and actions that reflect the challenges of change will emerge. One of the most gracious gifts we can give one another is the acknowledgement that we recognize a change someone is experiencing or that a change appears easy or difficult for someone. By reflecting what others are experiencing through

## CHOOSING A CONFLICT MANAGEMENT STYLE

In every situation we are responsible for our actions. Conflict situations offer each of us an opportunity to choose a style for responding to the conflict. The key to effective conflict prevention and management is to choose the conflict management style appropriate for the conflict. Most of us have a favorite style that we use in conflict situations, but we are all capable of choosing a different style when it is appropriate.

Five main types of conflict management styles are described here: cooperative problem solving, competing, compromising, avoiding, and accommodating. Animals are associated with each style to help you remember the differences. Remember that animals, like people, may have a favorite style, but they may also choose to adopt a new style in special situations.

## COOPERATIVE PROBLEM SOLVING

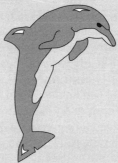

Choosing a cooperative problem-solving style enables people to work together so that everyone can win. People who use this style try to find a solution that will help everyone meet their interests and help everyone maintain a good relationship.

A dolphin usually chooses a cooperative problem-solving style. Dolphins use whistles and clicks to communicate with each other to catch food cooperatively and to summon help. For example, when a dolphin is sick or injured, other dolphins will help it to the surface so it can breathe.

Although the dolphin usually chooses to be a cooperative problem solver, it can also choose other styles depending on the situation. For example, if a shark is in the area, a dolphin with a baby will choose to use a competitive style to deal with the shark. Continuing to use the preferred style of cooperation would greatly endanger the life of the baby dolphin.

---

**Figure 1.4** Conflict response styles.

## COMPETING

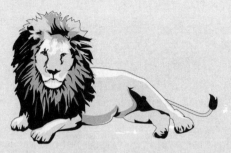

Choosing a competitive style means a person is putting his or her interests before anyone else's interests. In fact, sometimes people who use the competitive style try so hard to get what they want that they ruin friendships.

A lion can be a symbol of a competitive style. The lion's roar helps the lion satisfy its interests. For example, if the lion's family is hungry and needs food, the lion may use its strength to obtain food and loud roar to protect its family.

However, the lion can also choose to use a compromising or accommodating style when playing or resting with a lion cub.

## COMPROMISING

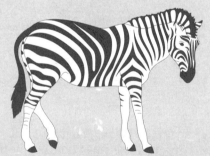

People choose a compromising style when it is important to satisfy some of their interests, but not all of them. People who compromise are likely to say, "Let's split the difference," or "Something is better than nothing."

A zebra can be a symbol for the compromising style. A zebra's unique look seems to indicate that it didn't care if it was a black horse or a white horse, so it "split the difference" and chose black and white stripes.

However, a zebra may not choose a compromising style for all things. A zebra may choose a cooperative or competitive style like the dolphin or lion depending on the situation.

*(continued)*

---

**Figure 1.4** *(continued)*

## AVOIDING

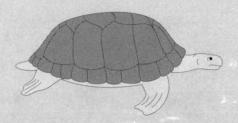

People who choose the avoiding style do not get involved in conflict. A person choosing the avoiding style might say, "You decide and leave me out of it."

A turtle is a symbol for the avoiding style because it can avoid everything by pulling its head and legs into its shell to get away from everyone else.

A turtle also chooses other styles at times. If it chose to always stay in its shell, it would miss out on everything from eating to swimming.

## ACCOMMODATING

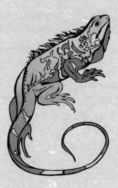

People who choose an accommodating style put their interests last and let others have what they want. Many times these people believe that keeping a good friendship is more important than anything else.

A chameleon is a symbol of the accommodating style because it changes its color to match the color of its environment. By changing its color, the chameleon fits quietly into its surroundings.

Although the chameleon may always change its color to accommodate its surroundings, it may choose other styles when it is hunting for food, taking care of its young, or hiding from enemies.

Reprinted, by permission, from T. Wheeler, 2004, *Choosing a conflict management style* (Columbus, OH: Ohio Commission for Dispute Resolution and Conflict Management).

**Figure 1.4**   *(continued)*

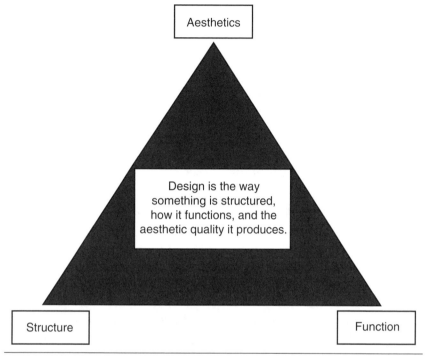

Aesthetics

Design is the way
something is structured,
how it functions, and the
aesthetic quality it produces.

Structure

Function

**Figure 1.5** Elements of design.

your gifts of words, or as a mirror to their feelings or actions, you can help support their metamorphosis into a well human being at a higher level of functioning.

As professionals who educate for health, we also need to know how to structure time for planned and sequential health instruction. Children and youth function best as learners when they are supported by a culture of wellness. As a result, their quality of learning is directly related to their quality of health. According to Ernest Boyer (1983), past president of the Carnegie Foundation, "Clearly no knowledge is more crucial than knowledge about health. Without it, no other life goal can be successfully achieved" (p. 304).

When the structure of your school schedule includes planned and consistent health instruction and evidence-based health curricula, young people will know how to function in health-enhancing ways instead of misdirecting their social, emotional, intellectual, spiritual, and physical energy in unproductive ways. Energy cannot be created or destroyed, but it can be renewed each day if given the time and space to do so.

In the following chapters you will be encouraged to develop your philosophy and pedagogy as a human being who is called to educate for health. Health is not opposed by disease but emerges out of the paradox of wellness and illness. None of us is perfectly formed, and few of us can claim an identity untouched by pain and pressure at the crossroads of daily living, where our private, personal, and public lives intersect. In this context, *private* means that only you and your Maker are privy to your identity formation; *personal* means you are part of the human race but custom-made for the journey; and *public* means you are part of a larger culture and society, with commonalities and differences that emerge in a dynamic story of life.

## CHAPTER FEATURES

### Principles of Practice

- Your thoughts, feelings, and actions as a professional form an integrative pattern of well-being that contributes to culture and helps others learn and live in that culture.

- Your identity is structured by your physical being, emotional being, intellectual being, spiritual being, and social being so that you can function as a human being. The quality of your life is determined by your private, personal, and public life experiences.

- When educating for health, your philosophy informs your pedagogy. The tension between the two can energize your theory and practice so they are productive—not destructive or reductive—for young people.

- Your educational philosophy is who you are and what you know. Your educational pedagogy is what you do with who you are.

- Change emerges from personal energy that has positive and negative effects. The tension between daily stress and conflict leads to change, also known as metamorphosis. This tension—or energy—can be perceived as positive, negative, or neutral.

- Change is the energy that emerges out of stress and conflict in the curriculum of life. Health, the curriculum of life, transcends disciplinary boundaries.

### Teacher Voices

An educator reflects on a philosophy of learning and teaching:

I believe that my journey to educate for health begins with who I am as a human being, guided by what I do with my gifts and talents. As an educator, I have a philosophy of learning that is tied to my personal identity. My philosophy is in continual transition as I learn more about how other people learn and what new pedagogies (and technologies) are available. My philosophy of learning is the foundation for my evolving philosophy of teaching. I integrate my philosophy and pedagogy to form my teaching platform. I also integrate my personal and professional stories to contribute to the profession of health education. I believe there are many pathways to identity formation; I also believe there are pathways that are marked by footprints and fingerprints unique to me. Each day that I am on the journey to educate for health, I have the ability to give voice to my calling, my questions, and my concerns. Discerning when to talk, when to listen, and when and how to respond continues to take me deeper into my vocation. Finding the invocation to my calling to teach and to write has been enhanced by the development of an avocation when I am not working. The relationship between my vocation, my avocation, and my invocation has transformed my life. To share that with others in community is a way to make a difference in the world.

*Valerie A. Ubbes, PhD, CHES;*
*associate professor and health educator; Miami University*

## Seeds of Growth:
## Signs, Symbols, and Patterns of Living and Learning

1.  Count the number of words in this chapter that use the prefix *inter*. What personal or professional ideas did you uncover in this word study? What pattern for life or for learning does that illuminate for you? Record your findings in your learning journal.

2.  Collect photos or film clips of children's faces when they are experiencing or reacting to a threatening situation. What does a response to danger look like? sound like? feel like? as you view the situation through the senses of a child or adolescent? What does a response to comfort look like? sound like? feel like? compared to a response to danger? Be sure to document your sources.

3.  In your learning journal, list your personal responses (e.g., hugs, bottled water, referral to a school nurse) to children and youth who are in need of health education or health care. In what areas of health or wellness do you feel competent? In what areas do you need professional development?

4.  In your learning journal, write a reflection on Palmer's (1998) statement about teaching well:

> In fact, knowing my students and my subject depends heavily on self-knowledge. When I do not know myself, I cannot know who my students are. I will see them through a glass darkly, in the shadows of my unexamined life—and when I cannot see them clearly, I cannot teach them well. (p. 2)

## Web Links for Living and Learning

Go online to the Children's Picture Book Database at Miami University (www. lib.muohio.edu/pictbks). Look for picture books that include keywords for health, five senses, safety, exercise, nutrition, hygiene, relationships, and sleep. Also do a Boolean search that combines one of these keywords with the keyword *multicultural* or the keyword for a specific culture. Select a representative sample of books from which to design "literature links" lessons for life for a diverse population.

## Books for Living and Learning

In his picture book *The Three Questions,* Jon Muth (2002) asks these questions: "When is the best time to do things? Who is the most important one? And what is the right thing to do?" Read about how a young boy, Nikolai, visits with his friends to uncover the meaning of these questions. Think of a situation where these questions were answered for you in your life in a similar way. Tell your story to another young professional and share how you plan to use this experience when you educate for health.

# 2

# Ways to Be:
# An Ontological Study

As the physicist Paul Gailey suggests, health can be described as the cooperation between cells and disease as the breakdown of cooperation. A cancer cell, for example, ceases to relate with other cells. For cancer cells replicate themselves at all costs: me, me, me and more of me. Cancer cells feed by eating other cells. They are the most ferocious example of a part living at the expense of the whole.

© by Mark Nepo, *The Exquisite Risk: Daring to Live an Authentic Life,* 2005

After reading this text, what will you know and be able to do? This text will help you educate for health and tailor health messages and instructional lessons for preK-8 learners. Why is this important? Health education that is communicated and directed to the learner can increase the likelihood of academic success in the school curriculum and enable young people to practice health-related skills, leading to an increased quality of life.

Before we can explore your professional story of what you will know and be able to do in educating for health, it is important that you take a journey into ways to be a human being. Ontology is a branch of philosophy that deals with the nature of being. As human beings, our origin and development follow a reasonably predictable path of growth and change. That is, we are all growing, changing, adapting, and aging each day as we function and live on earth.

Even though as a young professional you may lack concrete examples about your career, the curriculum of life is grounded in who you are now in a world of change. Until you can recognize and capture your own story of life within the bigger order of change, you will lack the direction you need for making important life choices. Although each day represents a small but important step in your final life journey, each day's experiences contribute to your identity formation. The ability to distinguish and interpret your direction along many possible choices, both personally and professionally, is found inwardly at the core of your identity. However, to journey into the core of your identity, you need to be in community with other learners and citizens of the world. We learn who we are while in the company of other human beings. We also learn who we are by being mindful of our unique gifts and talents in a daily journey of identity formation.

In the story *Seven Blind Mice*, author Ed Young (1992) illustrates seven possibilities for seeing a certain object through the lived experiences of seven blind mice. Each mouse explores the object by going on a trip to visit and discern what that certain something is. After experiencing the object, each mouse claims a different perspective by naming the object from that day's journey. After six days, the seven mice, still in community and open to the perspectives of others, are now rich with the collective interpretation of the same object. Not one of their perspectives is the same; each mouse claims a different object. On the final day, the seventh mouse starts on her journey. She runs up one side and down the other; she runs across the top from end to end. Building on the background knowledge of her lived experience with her companions during the week, she suggests that the object is not six different things but the whole of an elephant. The story ends with a powerful insight: "Wisdom comes from seeing the whole." The seventh mouse could not have uncovered this truth without the company of others and their points of view.

From your place in the world, you may be seeking clarity about how your personal and professional lives weave a story for your life. It is important that you take time to reflect on your role as a human being first, including reviewing your unique gifts and talents. The educational literature suggests that if we are to increase the chance of student success in classrooms, we need a highly qualified teacher leading that educational experience. That means you will need to know who you are as a human being at your core, then add additional layers of what you know and what you do outward from your core.

## Observing Children as Human Beings

If you ever watch a child sleeping, there is peacefulness in the quiet of his rest. You can see the rise and fall of his chest during breathing. And if you are close enough, you may hear his heartbeat with your ears or feel his heartbeat with your gentle touch on the inside of his wrist.

The pulse of the arteries beneath his skin and yours originates from deep inside the chest cavity, where cardiac muscle maintains a steady beat of electrical signals. A chemical interaction of sodium and potassium, two basic elements of chemistry also found inside the human body, creates an electrochemical potential that gives the heart tissue a source of power. Without this potential energy, the heart would stop pulsing and the blood would stop flowing between the body, heart, and lungs, thus leaving the child without a fresh supply of oxygen to sustain his life.

During the child's sleep, his brain functions with electrochemical rhythms similar to those in his heart. An electroencephalograph detects the action potentials via electrodes on his scalp. An electrocardiograph does a similar detection of the action potentials of his heart. Although your own hand on the child's head cannot detect the delta waves while he sleeps, different brain waves are patterned as alpha, beta, and theta depending on his mental activity during consciousness. Once awake and moving about his day, the young child can be noted as a "live wire" or "full of energy," thus emphasizing his intense emotional excitement and the suitable analogy to the electricity that powers his body and brain.

The dynamics between rest, sleep, and play are in continuous motion for all human beings. Whether asleep or awake, our bodies sustain a changing rhythm of life that is cyclic and vital. Sometimes we lose sight of the inside energy of our bodies working on our behalf. The body's design is a fabulous interaction of structures (bones, muscles, nerves, organs) that function as 10 body systems within one organism. Certain organs such as the medulla oblongata control respiration, circulation, and other bodily functions. Have you ever thought about your medulla oblongata, which sustains your life? Do you even know what it looks like or where it is located in the lower portion of the vertebrate brain?

How often have you appreciated the ions that are really in "charge" of your life, forming molecules and nutrients for living?

When a baby is born, we take delight in her eyes, nose, mouth, ears, fingers, and toes; in the color and softness of her skin; and in the color and amount of hair on her head. Because the baby cannot communicate in the spoken word until later, we admire and carefully watch the expression in her eyes, the changes in her nose and mouth, and the ways she grasps her fingers or wiggles her toes. We eventually teach these body parts to toddlers as they learn to speak, and we move on to naming the clothes that cover these body parts. By puberty, these body parts go through even more changes, some by choice (e.g., hairstyles, makeup, body art). In health education, we even begin to move inside the body to name organs and systems. Since children and preteens are still very concrete learners, the inside of the body doesn't make much sense to them unless they can learn in concrete ways through models and movies. For the most part, it may be premature to teach younger children about the inner workings of the human body.

## Ways to Be

The U.S. Army had a jingle on television that promoted confidence in the identity of youth: Be all you can be . . . in the army. The notion of being who you are is essential in all learning. Too often in social situations, we jump quickly to the proverbial question "What do you do?" Such a phrase is rarely used on children and youth until graduation from high school or university. However, even before that time, the inquiry takes a more subtle form: What do you want to *do* when you grow up? Sometimes the question is asked closer to the core: What do you want to *be* when you grow up? A more freeing and promising inquiry is grounded in the question *Who* do you want to be? And an even more essential question supports growth like no other: Who are you right now?

If we were to analyze what human beings were meant to *be*, we would honor the various dimensions of our health as essential to our wellness. Sound health integrates the five dimensions of health into the concept of wellness, which means wholeness. A surplus of one dimension of health cannot make up for the lack of another; each dimension forms the whole. Specifically, human beings were not meant to be hungry (need food), tired (need sleep), lonely (need relationships), bored (need play), thirsty (need drink), or afraid (need safety). When these needs reveal themselves in life, we must seek ways to meet our intrapersonal (self) and interpersonal (social) requirements.

As a professional who educates for health, you need to pay attention to the children and youth under your care. Begin each day with a greeting and interaction that lets you get a sense of each learner in your classroom. Throughout the first 20 minutes, encourage each person to focus on your plans for the day and to be attentive to what, when, why, how, and where you want to take the class for the learning session. Rather than launch right into the learning episode, you might observe the face and body language of each person as you speak, scanning the entire class for cues to individual needs.

To emphasize their goals for the lesson, effective teachers use tactics such as the following: "Okay, can someone please state the first thing we are going to do when I stop talking? What is the next thing you heard? And then, what is our final goal by the end of this session? Great! Does anyone have any questions or comments?" These cues to action can get a group of people to respond in a collective way.

As a professional who educates for health, be mindful of your learners' patterns of action, and take note of which children are energized to move into the journey you have outlined and which children are reluctant to get involved. Teachers cannot truly know each student daily. Just because a student is slow to move into action does not mean he is trying to be uncooperative. It may mean he is dealing with an issue that happened on the way to school or something that happened the night before at home. Teachers are sometimes too quick to ask the question "How are you?" and assume the responder will be honest and open on the first prompt. Many times, it takes a slower pace—perhaps evident later in the lesson—for a student to find the space to disclose verbal or nonverbal information to his teacher.

A professional friend once told me a story about her own son, who was continually being cued by the teacher to sit down and pay attention. The teacher was a fast-paced, efficient woman who was highly organized and eager to teach her lessons. Because it was early in the school year, the third-grade boy was still responding in the classroom with some of his second-grade tendencies, namely his habit of moving from table to table to see and talk to his classmates. The teacher called my friend and asked whether her son was hyperactive at home and constantly needing reminders. The mother was dumbfounded. Her son was bright and generally obedient, needing only occasional cues to follow directions. After several phone calls about this issue, my friend called her son's second-grade teacher to ask if this was a problem the year before. The second-grade teacher said the little boy often showed a pattern of caring for his classmates that at first notice looked as if he was just out of his seat a lot. In fact, it took at least two months before the second-grade teacher took the time to just sit and observe his actions. The bottom line was that my friend's son tended to be socially sensitive to his second-grade classmates at the start of each day, especially during different transitions. The teacher learned to read the bodily actions and verbal messages of this boy, who moved about her classroom emotionally healing others and touching those who were quiet and less social.

In this true story, the third-grade teacher focused more on teaching her subject matter than on attending to her students' personalities. There are times for both, and children need to learn when it is appropriate to focus on relationships (social health), feelings (emotional health), and academic tasks (intellectual health). If only these dimensions of health could be integrated in a more holistic way in schools. As a young professional, you will need to balance the needs and interests of children with the policies and demands of the curriculum.

When children experience a curriculum that takes center stage each day, they grow up disliking schooling because the curriculum is not connected to who they are. Children are egocentric and seek ways to meet their social, intellectual, physical, emotional, and spiritual needs. As they sense the sights, sounds, smells, tastes, and touches of life and interpret them from personal experience, they respond to the world in their own unique ways. A wise teacher will be the facilitator between the student and the curriculum, balancing a fine boundary line for children to cross and travel and explore from their own experiences. This is what is meant by giving children access to the curriculum and not traveling the road for them. You should also resist the urge to be a tour guide, telling students how to experience the curriculum.

So what might be a reasonable goal each day as you begin teaching? Begin each day with the reminder that you are called to educate, and then be thankful for that calling to be who you are. You will spend an incredible amount of time putting structures and guidelines in place, then facilitating others to work within those guidelines. This conforming structure is important when teaching groups of people so that each person can gain access to the lesson and accomplish its goals. However, a wise teacher will also be sensitive to requests from students who want to do something a little differently or try something outside the structures of your plan. This flexibility works best after you have come to know your students a little better. This type of education is called differentiated instruction. By recognizing that each learner has different needs at different times, you can learn to differentiate your educational goals so that you help learners access the information in their preferred learning style.

## Learning Styles

If you are the type of learner who likes to follow a script and be organized from start to finish, you might begin your teaching career with that same expectation of your students. If you like to talk things out with colleagues before you begin teaching, you might encourage this in your students by allowing small-group work or whole-class discussions. If you like to think deeply about why certain things work and prefer to study new approaches supported by evidence, you might expect your students to discover and learn in the same way. If you like to think about ideas and make new connections as you learn, you might expect your students to be seekers of information as well. Each of these preferences is a way that people like to learn. You will probably try to build them into your planning and teaching patterns. This is a developmental way for you to connect the curriculum to individual learning preferences.

According to Gregory and Chapman (2002), "Teachers must make every effort to know learners in order to meet their diverse needs. Just as clothing designers must know about the many fabrics and styles to create a garment to suit the wearer, so in classrooms we teachers must know about our learners so that we may find the strengths and unique-ness of each child" (p. v). Learning styles are one way to identify your learning preferences as well as those of your learners.

As an educator, you will prefer to use certain interpretations or styles when gathering information for your teaching and learning, and your ways of accessing information are often unique to you. Recently, I gave a presentation in Atlanta on multiple forms of information. A middle-aged man raised his hand halfway through my presentation to ask about my use of a star to represent our human senses. I explained my rationale and then offered my reason for liking the symbol of a star. I suggested that if he were to cut an apple in half on the transverse axis, he would find a star in both halves of the apple. I hoped that my abstract, symbolic use of a star represented a more concrete example for him. According to Strong, Silver, and Perini (2001), the mastery learner emphasizes memorization and looks for specific knowledge and skills to be learned. A mastery learner performs as a competent worker and values correct-ness and competence.

As an experienced educator, I have a decent competence in all four learning styles, but my preference is to be more abstract and concep-tual and not as concrete. For example, as an understanding learner, I emphasize reasoning in my work and value critical thinking and problem solving. I tend to look for ideas, patterns, principles, and rules in my learning. The fact that I do thought experiments on a weekly basis by thinking of ways to organize and look for patterns in information makes me a complex thinker.

Strong, Silver, and Perini (2001) promote two additional learning styles known as interpersonal and self-expressive. They are similar because the learner likes to feel in subjective ways, which is in contrast to the two learning styles just mentioned that involve thinking in objective ways. Of the interpersonal and self-expressive styles, the first is more concrete and the latter is more abstract. So since I enjoy teaching through patterns, I must point out that the understanding learner and the self-expressive learner are both abstract learners (which by reasoning makes the mastery learner and interpersonal learner both concrete learners).

For fear that I may have already isolated some of you from understanding the different learning styles, I direct you to table 2.1 so you can see a more useful way of representing learning styles—that is, by seeking patterns of similarities and differences across the rows and between the columns. Learning styles can also be analogous to "windows of opportunity" (Silver, Strong, & Perini, 2000), with four boxes representing four different points of view or perspectives. Since I am also a self-expressive learner, I like to emphasize this inventive approach to learning styles by performing as a creative contributor. When you read through the rest of this chapter, you will see that I value philosophical issues and original products. Now that you know I like to access information as an understanding and self-expressive learner, you might be astute to ask what is the difference between my preferences to think in objective ways (understanding learner) and to feel in subjective ways (self-expressive learner). You will find the answers to that question in chapter 3, but for now I will tell you one last story of my excitement about learning styles.

I have been using learning styles in my teaching for about six years. Each semester, I assess my learners using an inventory so that I know what preferences they bring to my classes. This is important so that I can give students more access to the course. One day as I opened my 15-minute presentation on learning styles with a PowerPoint, drawings on the board, and lots of questions and discussion, a student raised her hand to ask, "What do you mean by access to information?" I was so happy that she asked, felt safe to ask, and wanted to know about that phrase.

By the next class period, I had my creative response in the form of photographs. What were the photos of? Well, they were pictures of the gates, doors, and bridges of the world. Since she was probably a concrete learner—and she was dealing with me as a more abstract learner—I used my self-expressive learning style to show pictures of concrete objects that represent the concept of access. This concept of access is very important

## Table 2.1  Learning Styles: Ways We Access Information

| Mastery learner | Interpersonal learner |
|---|---|
| Likes to gather information by human senses in *concrete* ways and by thinking in *objective* ways | Likes to gather information by human senses in *concrete* ways and by feeling in *subjective* ways |
| **Understanding learner** | **Self-expressive learner** |
| Likes to gather information by intuition in *abstract* ways and by thinking in *objective* ways | Likes to gather information by intuition in *abstract* ways and by feeling in *subjective* ways |

Adapted, by permission, from H.F. Silver, R.W. Strong, and M.J. Perini, 2000, *So each may learn: Integrating learning styles and multiple intelligences* (Alexandria, VA: Association for Supervision and Curriculum Development), 22, 25. By permission of Ho-Ho-Kus, NJ: Silver & Strong Associates, LLC.

because when you educate for health, you will design lessons to help people with different learning styles get access to the health-related information that is valid and reliable. In our meeting of the minds at the crossroads between concrete and abstract, we met in the middle with a representation of something abstract (e.g., the concept of access) through the use of concrete objects (e.g., photos of gates, doors, and bridges). After that, I quickly moved my students into small cooperative groups so they could increase their opportunities for accessing information through their interpersonal learning styles. Learning styles increase the transparency of your teaching–learning plans as you purposely move across and between styles to give a variety of learners greater access to your lessons.

## Narratives of Experience

This book embarks on a narrative of experience. Each of us might think of "experience as the text" (Connelly & Clandinin, 1988, p. 198) because as you read, think, talk, and write about learning, you gain insights into your growth and development. As you author your story of teaching and the role that health will play in your personal and professional development, you will need to be ever mindful of your learners, who will need to give voice to their own personal stories of health and well-being.

I once had a student comment that she wished she were still learning under me. Although it surprised me to hear her say it in that way since I prefer to model a community of learners when I teach, "learning under me" was her way of showing me respect and saying that she came to deeper understanding as a person when we interacted in the classroom. After having this student in four different professional classes, our roots of understanding about the subject matter and each other grew deep beneath the surface. We had journeyed together and constructed several teaching–learning experiences beyond what either of us would have discovered alone. This same student was the first from my university to move her student-teaching internship to Camp Kern, a YMCA extended-classroom setting where fifth and sixth graders came to investigate life, learning, and health during a week-long camping experience. She was also the first of my students to take her talents into an international teaching commitment to Mongolia, where she taught all subjects to children of American doctors in a multi-age classroom. After several years, she returned to the United States to pursue her master's degree in public health.

The image of a large tree may be one way to think about your role as a teacher. Like a tree, your arms can stretch out to shadow and shade but also to protect and inspire what your learners will gain from your time together. The sunlight and climatic elements reach through your arms to the fingers of your students as they interact with you and with each other in a wide range of learning conditions and daily experiences. Seeds of cognitive knowledge are passed along through treelike branches during the teaching–learning cycle to generate new insights and growth.

With their stately boughs and arms, some oak trees keep their leaves through most of the winter and unfurl their new growth late in the spring. On late winter days I enjoy the pleasure of watching oak leaves dance across the top of snowdrifts near my library where I write. The cold winter wind moves the oak leaves with leaps and pauses in a rhythmic way as if to say, "We are dancing! We are dancing!" They stand on their stems to show their veins, arms, and legs with a reach of strength and promise. These same leaves remind me of vibrant red maple leaves in fall, colorful songbirds in springtime, and butterflies in summer moving in the breeze and expressing themselves like children in the classroom of different seasons. The birds and butterflies spread their wings to fly from tree to flower, just as children move from seat to seat, activity to activity, and classroom to classroom. You can certainly reflect on the past and dream of the future, but when you walk through the doors of a school, it is alive with the here and now—and your story is to be lived in the present tense.

## Your Voice Is a Part of the School's Vision

When you enter a school to teach and learn, it is always a good practice to read the vision and mission statements to get a sense of the community and collegiality of the people there. Schools have mission and vision statements about their plans for students so that all the professionals in the school will have a focused target to work toward during the year. You may be fortunate to help write or revise the vision and mission statements of the school in which you work. If so, you will probably draw on your personal practical knowledge because you will know what needs to be said about the nature of teaching and learning.

If you are a new teacher, it is important to pause and listen to the veteran words of your colleagues. But your ideas and insights are also very important in the dynamic culture of a school. Your voice should be heard, renewing the wisdom of the more experienced so that you all join together in community to make the school a healthy, vibrant place to work, to play, to learn. Your ability to share who you are with your professional colleagues in small groups and large groups is an important backdrop to how you establish the voice and choice of your students as a community of learners in your classroom.

## Human Beings First

By learning how to observe children, you will have more ideas about what they are interested in and how to plan for instruction. From a health and wellness perspective, it is also important to know the typical pattern of each child and adolescent so you can detect atypical patterns of behavior, such as what might occur with abuse or violence. The basic premise of identity formation is that we must look beneath the behaviors of children and youth to know their core well-being.

The way you model health-related skills and behaviors is a necessary prerequisite when educating children and youth about their personal health. They will look to you as a role model, for better or for worse, because you are a living, breathing human being that engages their sensory awareness and curiosity, probably more than a planned lesson about health. Eventually, we can move these young people from personal to public awareness, even a global perspective, but we must start with self-awareness and understanding. That is why I begin at the same place with you.

## Personal Practical Knowledge

I have chosen to draw on my personal practical knowledge when writing this book because my narrative of experience can model for you how a teacher can practice the skills of reading, reflecting, and writing. My story unfolds out of my commitment to educational inquiry that embraces pedagogy as a cornerstone for health education.

All health educators, like teachers of any discipline, must be able to move beyond "teaching as telling" to educating people to access information through multiple language forms, formats, and channels. In educating for health, you will also draw on a rich repertoire of pedagogical strategies. However, the focus should be on the people (learners) first, then on drawing out, selecting, and tailoring the content and messages to fit the learners.

Elliot Eisner, a noted curriculum scholar in arts education, suggests that narratives are a good way to reflect on teaching practices. Eisner (in Connelly & Clandinin, 1988, p. x) cautions us about their acceptance by some educational scholars but highlights why they are important:

> The metaphors by which teachers live, the way they construe their work, and the stories they recount tell us more profoundly about what is going on in their lives as professionals than any measured behavior is likely to reveal. But to use such data one must have courage. Narratives are regarded as "soft," and soft data do not inspire confidence among the tough-minded. . . . The willingness to pursue these elusive but informative aspects of educational life is not common within a framework that seeks "best methods" and measured outcomes.

## Other Places to Educate for Health

As you develop your narrative of experience, you should broaden your scope of where you will educate for health. You can start with health education in schools, then extend health-promoting messages to other places. Because parents and extended family members likely received limited health education when they went to school, children may not get the guidance they need through positive health-related messages from home to school and into the community. Too few adults model healthful lifestyles and tell informed stories about health. And that includes current teachers who may not have received consistent preK-12 health education when they went to school.

Educating for health should occur both inside and outside the classrooms: in homes, in boardrooms, and at neighborhood block parties. In my middle school health education class, teacher candidates and health professionals are given the freedom to plan health lessons for youth on cruise ships, at museums, in after-school programs, in Boys & Girls Clubs, in faith-based institutions, and in prisons. Health education must move outward from homes and schools into the community and corporations so we can sustain a healthy citizenry. When we use that philosophy of educating for health (Allegrante & Sleet, 2004), we are drawing on the ecological model from public health.

## Ecological Model

The bigger story of human health and well-being is given shape through an ecological perspective. An ecological perspective within the biological sciences refers to the relationship between organisms and their environments. Within sociology, psychology, and public health, the ecological perspective refers to the interaction of humans with their physical and sociocultural contexts (Sallis & Owen, 1997). The discipline of health education emerges from the concepts of education and health. The goal of health education is to promote, maintain, and improve individual and community health (NCHEC, 1996).

The ecological model (Eddy, Donahue, Webster, & Bjornstad, 2002) from the public health literature has five elements that begin at a core microlevel and then move outward to a macrolevel of influence. These factors, shown in figure 2.1, include the following:

1. Intrapersonal factors, which include the knowledge, attitudes, beliefs, and personality traits of an individual
2. Interpersonal factors and processes of family, friends, and peers who may support or be role models to the individual

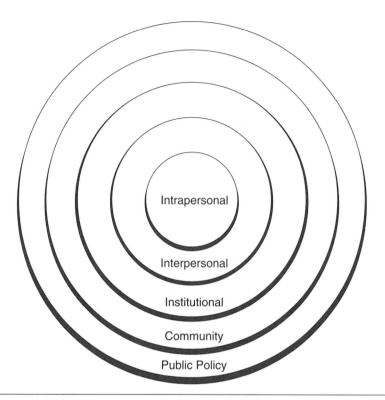

**Figure 2.1**　Ecological model.

Adapted, by permission, from J.M. Eddy et al., 2002, "Application of an ecological perspective in worksite health promotion: A review," *American Journal of Health Studies* 17(4): 197-202.

3. Institutional factors, which include rules, regulations, policies, and informal structures that may constrain or promote the recommended health behavior

4. Community factors, which exist as formal or informal social networks, norms, and standards in a location (e.g., neighborhood, state, region, nation, and world)

5. Public policies and laws that regulate or support healthy actions and practices for disease prevention, control, and management

The balancing act between individuals and their communities is a consistent theme in several educational models and theories. For example, Howard Gardner's theory of multiple intelligences (1993) promotes an intrapersonal intelligence and an interpersonal intelligence (Moran, Kornhaber, & Gardner, 2006). Lazear (2003) interprets these intelligences as being self smart and people smart. Ubbes (2004) labels these as intra-personal introspective (or I/I intelligence) and interpersonal social (or I/S intelligence). Learning styles theory (Silver, Strong, & Perini, 2000) names one of the four learning styles as interpersonal. Individuals with a preference for an interpersonal learning style like to access information through other people and are motivated by opportunities to learn about things that directly affect people's lives.

This text contributes to the health education literature because it brings three educational theories into health education—learning styles theory (chapter 2), multiple intelligences theory (chapter 4), and constructivist theory (chapters 3 and 5)—and into the core of the ecological model. In fact, the first two microlevels of the ecological model address how individuals and groups of people interact within the macrolevels known as place-based environments (e.g., institutions and communities). Policies structure the places and people of the ecological model in an ecosystem. Policies are ideological products made by professionals working alone and together within different institutions and communities to influence a plan or course of action.

McLeroy, Bibeau, Steckler, and Glanz (1988) first proposed an ecological model as a framework for planning health promotion programs from an educational and ecological perspective. Health professionals use the model to look at factors affecting health-related behaviors and environments. Eddy and colleagues (2002) state the following:

> As a means to explain health behavior, the ecological approach forces one to look for the cause of a health issue or problem from multiple perspectives. For example, eating behavior may be a function of personal knowledge and attitudes about food (intrapersonal). But, it could also be influenced by peer pressure (interpersonal), healthy food choices in company vending machines (institutional), an ample supply of fresh fruits and vegetables in local groceries (community), and the availability of free or reduced price lunch in schools (public policy). (p. 197)

Eddy and colleagues (2002) have suggested other applications of the ecological model. In worksite smoking-cessation programs (including those in schools where teachers and administrators might smoke), health educators can offer educational programs to help smokers quit (intrapersonal factors); address the social issues related to smoking on the job (interpersonal factors); and examine worksite smoking places, institutional smoking policies, and community and state tobacco laws.

# Objective Versus Subjective Structures for Teaching and Learning

When you educate for health, you take people beyond learning about information, resources, and services to the point of using them in ways that are health enhancing. Sometimes we go to people and sometimes they come to us, but however they enter or exit the learning experience, we must be able to draw out their personal connection with the information. When that happens, the learning experience is said to be personally relevant, engaging, and transformational—it mattered to that person.

If we put ourselves at the center of the lesson and fail to invite our learners' stories, we will transform the learning experience for ourselves, but not give others access to their own capacity for transformation. If we put disciplinary content at the center of the lesson and fail to invite our learners' interpretations of those disciplinary stories, we will not engage learners beyond passive participation in the discipline. If we exclude rather than include stories and interpretations, we will not release the full capacity of the information. In the end, we must understand that information is "in formation," but it is up to each learner to make meaning of the forms, e.g., words, pictures, numbers, rhythms, body language, and environmental cues. Using information in health-enhancing ways invites a dynamic way of learning that is constantly changing and transforming one individual at a time in the world.

A colleague once explained that language in itself has no meaning until a person brings meaning to it through the mental process of cognition. That is, written words are just ink on a page and spoken words are vibrations of air until a person makes sense of them within the framework of his or her human experiences. This is how I explain and make meaning of his comment from my physiology and education backgrounds:

In the former example of written words, you need to translate them by seeing and decoding the signs and symbols on the page via sensory-motor pathways, then think and read the words into meaning through conscious cognitive actions. To understand the printed words is to comprehend the meaning and importance of the words in that context or circumstance.

In the latter example of spoken words, you need to translate them by hearing their sound waves and rhythms via sensory-motor pathways, then mindfully think about the spoken words with cognitive-behavioral responses. You will learn about cognitive-behavioral responses in chapter 4. However in this context, we can imagine that a person will use verbal responses and kinesthetic body language to respond to the spoken words. It is, of course, possible that the person will make no response whatsoever, leading to a breakdown in communication known as a knowledge gap.

Palmer (1998) suggests that learning emerges from two models of education known as the objectivist myth of knowing (figure 2.2) and the community of truth (figure 2.3). In the former, the object to be studied is "out there" in the world to be known, much like policies or facts or figures of the ecological model. People who are trained to know these objective truths are called experts; they access the information and share it with amateurs, who are not as knowledgeable or expert about the information. The schematic of figure 2.2 shows baffle lines from the object to the expert and from the expert to the amateurs to prevent the flow of knowledge from going back up. Only the expert "knows" and holds the key to objective knowing, and that is why Palmer calls this the objectivist myth of knowing.

When we educate for health, the community of truth (figure 2.3) may serve us and our learners in more health-enhancing ways. In this schematic, the web of influence includes a "conversation of learners" that

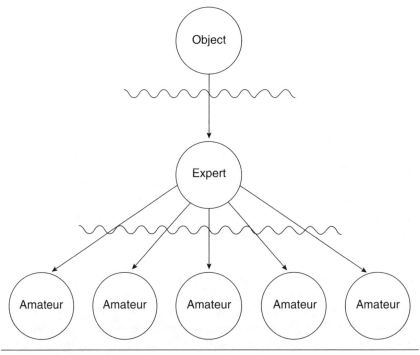

**Figure 2.2** The objectivist myth of knowing.

From P.J. Palmer, 1998, *The courage to teach* (San Francisco: Jossey-Bass), 100. Reprinted with permission of John Wiley & Sons, Inc.

honors the knowledge and perspectives of individuals from their place in the world. We come to know the subject at the core of the network, while in relationship with one another and in relationship with the subject. The patterns and pathways of communication are multidimensional, multidirectional, and multirelational. The complexity of this communal circle gives human beings space to access the subject under consideration.

You may have a tendency to conclude that the objectivist and communal ways of knowing, teaching, and learning are in conflict with one another. However, this is not a necessary assumption. By keeping these schematics in your mind as schema for organizing your own understanding of education, you will have the infrastructure for sound decision making in different institutions and communities. By knowing Palmer's views and being flexible in your application of these models for your own life journey, you may be able to influence and construct safe and supportive environments for health promotion (Learning First Alliance, 2001).

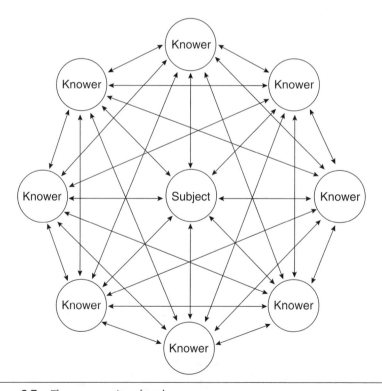

**Figure 2.3**   The community of truth.

From P.J. Palmer, 1998, *The courage to teach* (San Francisco: Jossey-Bass), 102. Reprinted with permission of John Wiley & Sons, Inc.

## Wellness, Well-Being, and Wellness Space

According to Greenberg (1985), health and wellness are conceptually different. Health has five components—social health, mental health, emotional health, spiritual health, and physical health—that are symmetrical in size and shape (figure 2.4). He states: "Wellness is the integration of the components of health into a meaningful whole; high level wellness is achieving a balance in this integration. Balance means that, as people work to improve one aspect of their health, they also need to work to improve others" (p. 5).

Like many others, I often use an apple to represent good health, supported by the phrase "an apple a day keeps the doctor away." As an exercise in critical and creative thinking, I often ask students to talk about the apple as a symbol of physical health, social health, intellectual health, and so forth (Ubbes, Hall, & Falk, 2004, pp. 9, 35-36), then to imagine the apple as a whole—even with its blemishes, dents, and bruises. As a metaphor for human wellness, the apple highlights that we cannot have perfect health, but we can still shine on the "outside" if we define ourselves by wellness rather than by only a few components of our health.

Once I decided to re-*search* the inner core of an apple by making a cross-sectional cut through its transverse axis. Many of you know that a star is exposed on the inside of the apple when you do this. Many do not know that the individual compartments containing the seeds are

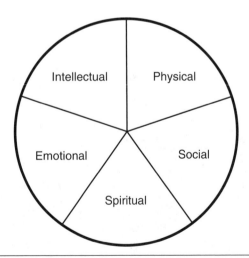

**Figure 2.4**   The wellness model.

Greenberg JS. Health and Wellness: A Conceptual Differentiation. **Journal of School Health.** Vol. 55, No. 10, p. 405. December 1985. Reprinted with permission. American School Health Association, Kent, Ohio.

surrounded by 10 faint dots in a circle around the star. It was a remarkable day of discovery for me when I did a deeper thought experiment with the apple as a metaphor for health and wellness. I envisioned the 10 dots in the fleshy part of the apple as representating the 10 human body systems and the five star compartments as representing the five human senses. Since the apple is a physical object, I guess I was thinking of my body as a physical being that could be explained in a concrete way through a comparison.

Next, I drew a picture of a star surrounded by 10 dots on a piece of paper, then connected the dots so that I had a diagram of a star surrounded by a circle. Five projected light rays emanated from the points of the star, which touched the circle in a coordinated way. This image resulted in five triangle shapes that reminded me of the wellness model (Greenberg, 1985) I had taught for years. This gave me a concrete model for conceptualizing the human body with its human senses. I reasoned that until we are fully aware of who we are and how we access information in the world through our human senses, we may not have the developmental readiness to conceptualize the wellness model. The star did not symbolize the wellness model to me, but the space around it did. This makes sense because the wellness model is an abstract concept that needs to be taught concretely. In some respects, it requires enlightenment (e.g., spiritual or intellectual insight) via the pathways of the human senses to be able to concretely sense and then think abstractly about our daily lives as having multiple dimensions of well-being.

In figure 2.5, I show the symbol of a star as a concrete object for labeling our human senses. The human senses of sight, sound, smell, taste, and touch are made possible by the physical structures of our eyes, ears, nose, mouth, and skin, respectively. The physical structures of these body parts help us function and communicate in the world. But our human senses have a two-dimensional story (and more). For example, our eyes can see in light and in darkness; our ears can hear and help us with equilibrium and balance; our nose can help us to smell and to breathe; our tongue can help us to taste and to talk; and our skin can help us with touch and knowing body positions and locations. As we educate for health, early childhood curricula should promote one function of each of the human senses, and middle childhood curricula should promote the second function of each. This age-appropriate developmental approach to the human senses can then be extended into ninth grade and beyond as we introduce additional functions of the human senses, including intersensory responses. Once learners have transitioned from concrete operational thinking to formal operational reasoning (Piaget, 1983), we can also promote the abstract concept of wellness, which gives us a mental framework for assessing our five dimensions of health each day. Developmentally, we can learn how to combine two or more health

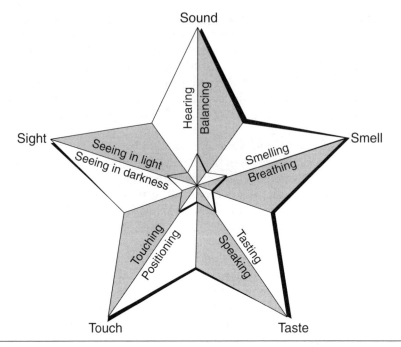

**Figure 2.5**   Human senses.

dimensions at the same time in order to work on the skill of integration that Greenberg promotes.

I later decided to refine my apple model even more so that it was developmentally appropriate for middle school youth. During the writing of this book, my own children spanned the years of 9 to 14, so I was acutely aware of their changes in response to health-related messages at home. Basically, my husband and I had to increase our cuing of health behaviors and reteach basic health skills even though our children had modeled consistent habits in their childhood. Although it was often frustrating for both the children and adults in our home, we continued to negotiate these changing times. Concurrently, I had to explain this phenomenon to college students who were enrolled in my middle childhood health education course ("Wellness Perspectives for Adolescents"). As a result, figure 2.5 evolved into a model called the wellness space of human well-being (see figure 2.6), with the goal of giving young people access to their multiple dimensions of health. I knew as a mother and as an educator that one must allow children to access information rather than drop it down their throats like a robin feeding worms to her hungry fledglings.

Through trial and error, I learned the value of giving space to my children, but I often overcued them: "How many servings of milk did you have today?" "Did you brush your teeth?" "Did you get enough sleep?" "Did you wash your hands?" "Did you say your prayers?" "Do you have your homework done?" "Did you thank Dad for driving you to school?" "Did you talk to your teacher?" These questions were my attempt to keep my children on the pathways to good health and well-being. I do know that children and adolescents face numerous choices on a daily basis, just as adults do. And the road to their enlightenment and "response-abilities" requires a personal awareness that comes from a raised consciousness. I believe the human senses are pathways that must be stimulated in a variety of ways in order for the road to widen toward wellness.

In summary, on a daily basis, humans have access to their physical, intellectual, emotional, spiritual, and social beings. The wellness space of human well-being model (figure 2.6) assumes that humans need space in their lives to gain access to their multiple dimensions of health. A closed environment with limited personal space, time, and energy for intellectual, social, and physical expression (to name a few) will play a determining role in your sense of well-being for that day. The best part of the well-being model is that you begin your journey anew every day.

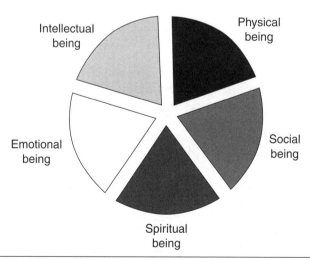

**Figure 2.6**   Wellness space of human well-being model.

# Hierarchies and Networks Inform Our Work

When they enter the medical field as professionals, doctors take the Hippocratic oath, which states that they will do no harm to their patients. Such a human-focused affirmation establishes a daily reminder for the physicians to serve their patients. This respectful oath treats humans with subjectivity rather than as objects to be known. You may recall a time when a doctor or medical specialist treated you with a distant objectivity without asking for your input. A neurologist I know would call that medical professional a doctor but would refer to a more interactive professional as a physician. This may be analogous to the distinction between a teacher and an educator. The word *educator* comes from the Latin word *educare*, meaning to bring to an understanding.

I usually tell my students that I appreciate the respect they afford me when I am a sage on the stage. As a professor, I have lots of philosophical and professional expertise to share with my students. On those days, I attempt to model how my personal and professional stories are interrelated—almost imagining myself as a tour guide to what's possible in the field. However, as an educator, I also find ways to invite my students into the storytelling. My students' journeys at Miami University, and your own collegiate journey wherever you are, play an important role in framing the stories of the discipline. You must come to know and then be able to communicate and practice the language and lessons of health education while in community with one another and with me. The integrative patterns of an expert's hierarchy in tandem with a communal network of knowers enrich and engage my interactions with students and the subject matter.

Although a teacher cannot truly come to know each of his students in a deep way, sometimes certain students choose to cross real or imaginary boundaries to talk to their teachers. Interactions that are student led and sought are some of the most meaningful of the teaching life. When a student goes out of her way to stay after class or speak in public with her teacher, both the teacher and the student benefit. Sometimes it is important for the teacher to cross personal boundaries to support or redirect a student toward health and safety. I do this whenever I see a person has ignored vital connections with his or her soul.

At a summer camp where I coached young gymnasts, I observed a daily pattern of mental and physical fatigue in a girl who kept trying a skill over and over with little success. I suggested that she listen to her body cues and do no further self-harm. Her response was surprising; she admitted no fatigue and continued to participate in training activities over the afternoon and evening sessions. The next morning the student arrived to class with extra bracing and tape on her wrists and ankles. Because she did not heed my suggestions about her need for rest, food, and water, she was no longer able to function. The structure of her body had weakened under the pressures of her goals. I was in a good position to give my student objective feedback because I saw her in class each day at the same time of the morning and did not directly observe her at other times when she worked on her training goals.

That morning, we sat down and reconsidered her daily goal so that she was still able to make incremental progress toward her weekly goal in my class. Remaining only as a guide on the side would not have worked in this teaching scenario. Instead, my expertise as a veteran gymnastics coach and my career as an educator combined to influence who I was as a human being, allowing me to sense the present and future needs of my student. From my core of well-being, I then moved into her life space to share my knowledge about gymnastics and health. I supported my student-athlete "well" by giving her access to her own objective and subjective ways of knowing. Educating for health emerges from the core of well-being that connects us all as human beings.

We must learn to value and care for the environmental and cultural situations that sustain our growth and development, and learn to limit those environmental and cultural situations that hinder our growth and development. In your role as a teacher *and* an educator, you will learn how to design environmental and cultural contexts for teaching and learning. In the end, our goal is to help people function better throughout their lives in aesthetic ways.

In conclusion, the expert teacher can take her students on side trips and investigative journeys that entice the senses, engage the present moment, and interest the heart while stimulating the mind. When educating for health, the teacher brings the world of people, places, and things to a crossroads for analysis (reduction) and synthesis (construction) in a health-promoting context of wellness. When children and youth cross the road to disease, disorder, or discovery with their peers as tour guides, your lessons of health must redirect kids to safer roads and narrower passageways. When teachers, parents, and caregivers contribute to congested roadways, the learning environment is reduced to chaos and confusion. You must help establish a place and space of learning that promotes the journey of wellness within an ecological model that educates for health. We will revisit this possibility in chapter 5. In chapter 3, we move to an epistemological study on ways to think about education and health.

## CHAPTER FEATURES

### Principles of Practice

- Teaching and learning are reciprocal actions when educating for health. Highly qualified teachers focus on student learning as the basis for their pedagogical decisions.

- Questions about human beings are based on the philosophical study of ontology. Ontology looks at ways to be a human being.

- Learning styles help differentiate how learners access information, from concrete to abstract patterns of knowing and through subjective and objective points of view. Learning styles differentiate the diverse abilities of human beings to learn.

- When educating for health, models from both public health and public education form integrative patterns for teaching and learning. This text helps bridge the theoretical and practical gaps in health education, forming new pedagogical patterns as you educate for health.

- The ecological model from public health education uses systems thinking, beginning at the core with the intrapersonal and interpersonal levels of influence.

- The human senses are pathways from outside to inside the brain. They can be taught in a developmentally appropriate way during the early childhood and middle childhood years. The human senses are at the core of identity development and can be represented by a star with five points symbolizing sight, sound, smell, taste, and touch. Wellness, a more abstract concept, can be represented by a circle that surrounds our human senses and frames our daily well-being.

### Teacher Voices

A health education major reflects on choosing to be a teacher, followed by a reflection one month into student teaching.

Deciding to become an educational professional was a big decision for me. I had been out of school for 10 years and was now a family man. Although going back to school was tough, I am not sure I would change my path. I worked as a laborer in several different facets. I then moved on to become a manager at an automotive paint company. This experience helped shape my philosophy on education. I feel that everyone deserves a chance to go to college and should be encouraged to do so. This was not the case for me. School was never a high priority in my family. I had some good teachers along the way but none that stood out as mentors.

Going to school as a nontraditional student was difficult, and my grades reflected this. The past three semesters I have been able to attend college full-time, and my GPA has steadily increased. Having chosen the path I did has helped motivate me to working hard to educate young students in achieving their goals.

As for my own goals, I want to continue to grow as an educator and a student of life. I feel that you never stop learning and improving your knowledge and techniques. I would say that my life's ambition would be to strive to be the best that I can be for myself, my family, my students and my school.

One month into student teaching . . .

We had a young lady miss last week because her mother died, and I could only think what if we had discussed the stages of grief in class how this might have helped. We have conferences Thursday, and I have requested a few parents to schedule. I also started an intervention class that meets for 20 minutes after lunch. It is mandatory for some and open to all. The idea is to get students caught up on homework and help those who are struggling. I have about 20 students, and it appears to be working. On our last test we only had about 10 that did not pass. However we had 17 that received a 100 or above (food for thought). It is nice to see students get disappointed because they received only a 95% on a test. My experience in the classroom has been everything that I thought it would be and more. I feel the highs and lows of these kids' academic success. I am starting to feel the part. As Mr. Adkins says, I am their ambassador to success.

*Jon Bennett, Miami University Alumnus in Health Education, 2001*

## Seeds of Growth:
## Signs, Symbols, and Patterns of Living and Learning

1. In your learning journal, write a reflection on Palmer's statement about the value of a teacher: "In our rush to reform education, we have forgotten a simple truth: Reform will never be achieved by renewing appropriations, restructuring schools, rewriting curricula, and revising texts if we continue to demean and dishearten the human resource called the teacher on whom so much depends" (Palmer, 1998, p. 3).

2. In your learning journal, write a reflection on Nepo's statement on the interplay between wellness and illness: "We needed each other, and it was hard to tell who was ill and who was well, who was giving and who was getting. In the center of it, we just tumbled in an authentic embrace that saved us all" (Nepo, 2005, p. 27).

3. In your learning journal, reflect on the relationship between health and wholism and how the following quote by Ubbes (2004) fits your professional philosophy:

Did you know that the original word, *hal*, gave us the verb *helan*, meaning to heal? According to Lasher (2001), "Literally, to heal is to make whole. From the same root [word] came the root *health*—the state of being whole or healed—and *hale*—that which is whole. What makes all this most interesting is the other word that came from *hal*: originally *halig*, meaning wholeness, it comes down to us as the word *holy*." This explains why holistic, having to do with wholeness, is an important concept we need to know and understand at the deepest level if we are to become health educators. How can we truly "educate for health" if we, ourselves, are not clear about health and how to obtain it in our lives? (pp. 1-2).

## Web Links for Living and Learning

On June 30, 2004, the President signed Public Law 108-265, the Child Nutrition and WIC Reauthorization Act of 2004. The law states that each local educational agency participating in a program authorized by the Richard B. Russell National School Lunch Act or the Child Nutrition Act of 1966 shall establish a local school wellness policy by school year 2006.

Many state agencies and school districts have already recognized the need to assist their students by encouraging healthy eating and physical activity. The number of state agencies that have developed model wellness policies continues to grow. At the local level, over 31,000 schools have enrolled as Team Nutrition Schools and are striving to have an impact on their students' eating and physical activity behaviors.

In the classroom students are taught to eat healthfully and to be active, but they also need the opportunity to practice those behaviors. Wellness policies combine education with practice to create healthful school nutrition environments and encourage healthy behavior.

Access the following Web link to learn what the components are for a wellness policy in American schools: www.fns.usda.gov/tn/Healthy/wellnesspolicyrequirements.html.

For a comprehensive view of a sample wellness policy for nutrition education and physical activity, including safe and healthful environments, access this site: www.schoolnutrition.org/uploadedFiles/SchoolNutrition.org/Child_Nutrition/Local_School_Wellness_Policies/SNALocalWellnessPolicyGuidelinesFinal.pdf. Discuss additional programming that you would recommend for other health behaviors needed by children and youth in your local schools.

## Books for Living and Learning

Jamie Lee Curtis and Laura Cornell have written a book called *Is There Really a Human Race?* (2006). The Library of Congress entry for the book states the following: "While thinking about life as a race, a child wonders whether it is most important to finish first or to have fun along the way." Have you ever felt like a member of the human race in a foot race? Use this book as a feature of an interdisciplinary curriculum unit on quality of life in health, genetics in science, genealogy in social studies, athletic races in physical education, rhythm of life in music, and the etymology of the word *gene* in language arts. Structure your investigation so that students will function in both an expert and cooperative way of learning. Use print- and technology-based resources for an aesthetic and artistic experience in design.

# Ways to Think: An Epistemological Study

Yet we must be watchful, for we all suffer both the impulse to separate and own and the impulse to unify and belong. Just as our eyes shut and open repeatedly, we take things apart and put them together constantly.

© by Mark Nepo, *The Exquisite Risk: Daring to Live an Authentic Life*, 2005

Constructivist theory suggests that people actively build their own knowledge structures, known as schema, rather than receiving information from experts by default or by adoption. Information is "constructed" and organized in the mind of the user through a network of neural pathways in communication with different brain lobes and cortexes. Such pathways form a neural infrastructure of sensory-motor and cognitive-behavioral experiences that are in continual synergy and feedback. Human experiences—known as prior knowledge—are integrated with continuous neural information via sensory-motor pathways then are interpreted by the brain in the form of cognitive-behavioral performances. Perkins and Blythe (1994) refer to these performances as "performances of understanding" leading to mastery of a discipline or domain (Gardner, 1997/1999). Since knowledge is socially constructed, humans need to model the roles and responsibilities of living well and learning well. Indeed, humans are influenced by individuals and groups of people who are positive and negative role models. Hence, young people need multiple representations of real-life human models to form a rich schema of background knowledge for promoting health. Unfortunately, the converse is also true. Representations of poor human role models also form a rich schema of experiences to practice, often as negative health habits and high-risk behaviors. The role of a health educator is to help learners uncover any misconceptions and biases they may hold in their background knowledge about wellness and illness, while negotiating and giving learners access to additional topics, concepts, and skills. Educators who can support and guide young people through multiple experiences of health promotion via practice and rehearsal provide the richest opportunities for age-appropriate growth and development.

This chapter investigates a philosophical and pedagogical platform for bridging constructivist theory into health education. In its simplest form, philosophy is the love of learning, and pedagogy is the love of teaching. Both these stories are essential ways to form your identity as a teacher. However, I am not really writing a book about teaching, for to do so would be to tell you how to teach. I am not sure I can accomplish such a tall order even with the 30-plus years I've been on this journey of educating for health and well-being. I am convinced that although we all draw on the theories, models, principles, and pedagogies of education regardless of what we teach or who we teach, there will be subtle and sometimes drastic differences in how we choose to organize our thinking about the teaching life. Consequently, this is why to teach well and to be well require the freedom and the space in which to access the multiple identities of our physical being, social being, intellectual being, spiritual being, and emotional being. Your daily construction of wellness, with its multiple dimensions of health, allows you to adapt with healthy actions as a human being in a changing world.

Your ability to utilize your strengths and compensate for your weaknesses on any given day will be uniquely yours. As you learn to pair your weaknesses with your strengths, your wants with your needs, and your problems with your possibilities, you will gain wisdom and insight into your journey of life.

## Constructivist Theory

The epistemology, or theory of knowledge, that informs my teaching philosophy is constructivism. Constructivism is learner centered and teacher facilitated. In a constructivist approach, students engage their minds (and hands) in understanding and making meaning. Students construct and reconstruct what they know about a concept or a misconception by meaning making. Danielson (1996) offers the following:

> Constructivism holds that people's understanding of any concept depends entirely on their mental construction of that concept—that is, their experience in deriving that concept for themselves. Teachers can, of course, guide the process, but students must undertake and manage the process of developing an understanding for themselves. The constructivist approach makes explicit that different individuals, depending on their experiences, knowledge, and *their cognitive structures at the time* will understand a given presentation differently. Research shows that people remember an experience based on what their pre-existing knowledge and cognitive structures allow them to absorb—regardless of a teacher's intentions or the quality of an explanation. (p. 23)

A constructivist approach to teaching and learning stems from a long and respected tradition in cognitive psychology through the writings of Dewey (1902), Vygotsky (1978), and Piaget (1983). "Constructivism is collaborative; it uses inquiry and problem solving to look for patterns in the learning process. In the process of learning the information from multiple sources, learners will also do something with the information" (Danielson, 1996, p. 25). Working together, teachers and learners will investigate information from different perspectives, draw their own conclusions, and personalize the information. Young adults (like you) have a continuum to follow in constructing meaning about your identity, learning, and intellectual development in university classrooms. Baxter-Magolda (Magolda, 2001; Magolda & King, 2004) cites self-authorship as a central goal of higher education as learners move through absolute, transitional, independent, and contextual ways of knowing.

Constructivism supports pedagogical approaches that are flexible, adaptive, and relevant to learners who help gather and generate information in collaborative discussions, solo and group investigations, and reflective writing. Subject matter remains important, but it is determined collaboratively through guided inquiry by teachers and learners during the learning process. To help learners improve how they think, "teaching has changed from covering the content to ensuring that students understand and know what they have learned. The switch has been to a less-is-more philosophy" (Halpern & Nummedal, 1995).

Constructivist theory suggests that learners construct and reconstruct information in order to learn (Brooks & Brooks, 1993). These constructions (and understandings) evolve when learners actively gather, generate, process, and personalize health-related information rather than passively receiving knowledge from teachers or health-related resources.

We can teach learners to organize existent and new information by using an inquiry-based pedagogy. Wurman (1989) claims that "knowing how things are organized is the key to understanding them" (p. 8). He offers these guiding questions for consideration:

How can I look at this information?

How would reorganizing the information change its meaning?

How can I arrange the information to shed new light on the problem?

How can I put the information in a different context?

When existing information is reorganized and connected in different ways, new patterns can lead to new meanings and interpretations. Consequently, a higher level of knowing results; this is called understanding.

Fahlberg and Fahlberg suggest that learners need help moving from individualistic, egocentric views of health and human potential to a community, sociocentric view of health and human potential. A more world-centric view brings a new "expanded self," with implications for optimal well-being (Fahlberg & Fahlberg, 1997). Even the National Health Education Standards recognize that learners in elementary, middle, and high schools need assistance in understanding personal, community, and global contexts about health. The eighth health education standard states that "students will demonstrate the ability to advocate for personal, family, and community health" (Joint Committee on National Health Education Standards, 2007, p. 8).

You can encourage your learners to be inquisitive about themselves and their world, but the kinds of questions they ask will depend on their developmental readiness. Younger children will usually ask questions about themselves; adolescents will begin to expand their worldviews, but their questions tend to stay within the parochial boundaries of peers as they relate to personal agendas, needs, and interests. Kids can be stretched to appreciate community and global concerns such as soup kitchens and rain forests and can certainly be taught to think about the well-being of people and their environments. However, you will need to offer more than an intellectualized account of the issues of hunger and the loss of medicines and food products from rain forests. Learning should result from personal, firsthand accounts through pedagogies of engagement. Such pedagogies include service learning, peer education, case studies, and cooperative learning.

The key to pedagogies of engagement is how learners are expected to interact with the subject matter. The constructivist process is dynamic and somewhat open-ended. For most learners, learning how to generate questions through problem posing and framing (Friere & Faundez, 1989; Shor, 1992) can be more instructive than knowing the answers.

King (1995) urges teachers to develop a habit of inquiry with their learners so they "can learn to ask thoughtful questions—of themselves and of each other" (p. 13). She continues:

> Good thinkers are always asking What does this mean? What is the nature of this? Is there another way to look at it? Why is this happening? What is the evidence for this? and How can I be sure? Asking questions such as these and using them to understand the world around us is what characterizes critical thinking. (p. 13)

You will need to cue and guide young learners with these questions until they are able to generate questions on their own (see table 3.1). By modeling a habit of inquiry, you will be encouraged when some of your learners follow your lead. And your learners can lead their peers into added discoveries and deeper investigations about the human body and brain, how they are designed, and how to promote an enhanced quality of life for self and others.

Some scholars argue that constructivism differs from behaviorism, the latter of which addresses how teachers teach (e.g., teacher behavior) and what students do to be healthy (e.g., health behavior). In health education, there is often a focus on what health-related behavior is accomplished. In my own classes, I often say, "We all know we are supposed to eat breakfast, but how many of you actually ate breakfast today?" This is usually followed by a series of questions probing the intentions and rationales for breakfast as it relates to quality of life and learning.

When educating for health, you will want to know what health-related skills (e.g., habits of mind) and what health behaviors (e.g., habits of health) are being practiced for daily well-being. Since health educators do use a behaviorist viewpoint when focusing on habits of mind and habits of health, we must cautiously analyze what is suggested by this approach.

Table 3.1  **Inquiry Questions Asked by Youth**

| Question | Guidelines for adults |
|---|---|
| Who am I? | • Give them the freedom to explore their world. Only then can adolescents begin to answer this question. |
| Am I normal? | • Give them room to be like their peers. Fitting in with peers helps adolescents feel "normal."<br>• Monitor youth activities by using the four W questions:<br>  - Where are you going?<br>  - With whom are you going?<br>  - What are you doing?<br>  - When will you be home? |
| Am I competent? | • Assist adolescents with their problems and challenges, but do not solve them.<br>• Ask questions instead of telling, such as "What are some things you could do?"<br>• Guide but do not direct. |
| Am I lovable and loving? | Adolescents develop best when they have supportive families and community life that includes the following:<br>• Warmth and mutual respect<br>• Serious and lasting interest of parents and other adults<br>• Adult attention to the changes they are experiencing<br>• Clear standards regarding discipline and close supervision<br>• Communication of high expectations for achievement and ethical behavior<br>• Democratic ways of dealing with conflict |

Reprinted from ReCAPP—ETR Associates (Education, Training, & Research), www.etr.org/recapp.

Habits of mind is a construct coined by Costa and Kallick (2000) in a series of books on developmental thinking habits: discovering and exploring, activating and engaging, assessing and reporting, and integrating and sustaining. In this text, habits of mind refer to the cognitive thinking skills that young people learn in order to successfully demonstrate habits of health. For example, a sixth grader must know how to assert himself through communication skills (i.e., a habit of mind) when being bullied on the playground. Effective communication in the form of assertive words and body language has a good chance of leading to improved relationships (i.e., a habit of health). Or a first grader must know to set a goal (i.e., a habit of mind) to drink three glasses of milk or eat calcium-rich foods each day for improved diet and nutrition (i.e., a habit of health). In both of these examples, the habit of mind is a cognitive action leading to a behavioral action. These cognitive-behavioral actions take a great deal of practice for successful patterning to develop into a habit of mind and habit of health, respectively. Although young people can and do learn habits of health by being cued by parents, teachers, and health professionals, the transition periods into middle school between fifth and sixth grades appears to be a time when the habitual nature of health tends to wane.

Many parents bemoan the added responsibility of reteaching the basic manners and health habits that their children consistently practiced at an earlier age. In this relapse of health-related skills and behaviors such as brushing the teeth, covering sneezes with an elbow, and washing hands before and after meals, caregivers and teachers must be patient and ask questions of their 'tweens and teenagers. This cognitive cuing is important so that kids can learn to think for themselves. This period of transition can be a key time for constructivist teaching and learning approaches. However, it does seem to result in frustrated teachers, parents, and caregivers.

There is reason to believe that constructivist and behaviorist theories can be complementary approaches when educating for health. Costa and Lowery (1989) suggest that learners will demonstrate many behaviors when they have learned to think. These include more persistence in problem solving, less impulsiveness when answering, increased ability to listen with empathy, acceptance of ambiguities, improved self-assessments, improved questioning ability, improved transfer between learning and work situations, and increased metacognition.

In using constructivist approaches when educating for health, teachers do not view people mechanistically, reducing learners to behaviors that can be manipulated and controlled. Instead, the object of analysis in health education needs to include the voice of the learners, who are asked to explain the thinking behind their choices. Such an exercise may seem futile when your *why* questions of tweens and teens result in "I don't know" or "I have no idea." But when educating for health, you must model persistence as a habit of mind because it can be a cue to action for others. The abstract questioning cues *what, where, why, when,* and *with whom* can be addressed in concrete ways. For example, we can offer a choice of a variety of fruits (what) on cereal (where) or fruit for a snack during an after-school club (when) with friends (with whom), instead of choosing a candy bar with high fat and sugar content (why). These questioning cues help young people to practice and concretize their cognitive skills (i.e., habits of mind) for different health behaviors (i.e., habits of health) with assistance from adults in school, home, and community contexts. We will continue to discuss habits of mind and habits of health in chapter 4.

## Constructivism in Education

Effective designers are always interested in meeting human needs to solve a problem. To meet needs, a designer finds an opportunity for unity between a product and the people who can use the innovation. In teaching, this opportunity for unity can involve an exchange of ideas and information between teacher and learners in a co-construction of the curriculum. Teachers who incorporate peer learning, cooperative learning, problem-based learning, and service learning have focused their work on learning—a pattern that reaps incredible power for the participants. For example, in service learning, middle school youths can meet the needs of an agency, organization, or institution by serving its participants or clients. In such an arrangement, youths work alone or together to solve problems of need by engaging with people in a setting outside the classroom. In preparation for service learning, teachers often use cooperative learning to bring students together in the classroom to practice sharing information and ideas for health promotion and disease prevention.

To extend teaching and learning to new dimensions, school administrators can establish a supportive environment in which education and health professionals can talk and share. Teacher leaders who craft effective lessons or tailor their student assessments to reveal learning outcomes should be encouraged to share with their colleagues on a consistent basis. A planned opportunity to share a lesson or assessment with professional colleagues will improve the teaching–learning design in ways that boost the original work to a new level. Innovations are often generated in a private environment, but they must go public to be shared, used, and refined. To that end, there is a need for interaction between education and health professionals, because we learn who we are and what we do when personal and professional thinking intersect.

A teacher's private thinking is often secret on purpose. Reflection on the day's events can bring satisfaction or frustration, affirmation or condemnation. These moments are often captured in notes or journals to assist in personal meaning making. Sometimes conversations with family and friends help sort out what worked well and why and what needs refinement. Ultimately, your journey of refining your professional practice will be mediated by your thinking like a teacher of children and youth, like a health educator, and like a professional who educates for health.

## What Is Design?

Design, from the Latin word *designare*, means to mark out or define by artistic arrangement or by forming plans in the mind, usually in a skillful way. Synonyms for the word *design* include *intend* and *plan*. In fact, if something is planned "by design," it is done with deliberate intention and purpose. As a noun, a design is a plan, sketch, or arrangement of details. Domains are an excellent place to study design. For example, design is found in architecture, music, photography, landscaping, dance choreography, and education. In their book *Why Design?* Slafer and Cahill (1995) suggest that, "Design is most successful when the problem is fully analyzed" (p. 31).

To be an effective teacher in curriculum and instructional design, you will investigate two broad types of knowledge: declarative knowledge and procedural knowledge. Declarative knowledge includes facts, topics, concepts, generalizations, principles, models, and theories. Procedural knowledge includes skills, strategies, techniques, methods, procedures, and processes. These ways to think about what we know and do help us to organize lesson plans, unit plans, and curricula in health education (and in any other discipline). When facts, topics, concepts, and skills are arranged in a planned pattern for teaching and learning, design emerges. Lesson plans often consist of assignments so that students can practice similar elements of design. To show how assignments and design are related, notice that the word *sign* is embedded in both words. Understanding how to design assignments in health education so they are relevant and engaging to your developmental learners will be a consistent problem to solve each day when educating for health.

## Design as an Inquiry Process

Design is an ongoing inquiry process for teachers. You design a lesson before you teach it. Then when you implement your plan, you may find yourself making adaptations and improvements during and after the lesson so the plan is more refined for the next time. Since your student profiles and audiences differ from class to class, these changes in design are to be expected.

Some elements of design are constant, however. Your students will have memorable learning experiences when you use repeating patterns of light, color, sound, rhythm, and movement in interesting and novel ways. Your learners will certainly remember more when cued for action using their olfactory, gustatory, kinesthetic, visual, and auditory senses during learning episodes. When educating for health, the right mix of sensory patterns will make learning more engaging, evocative, and emotional.

You can also use patterns in words and pictures through the evidence-based instructional strategy of a metaphor. Berman and Brown (2000) suggest that "if a picture is worth a thousand words, then perhaps we can regard a metaphor as being 1000 pictures" (p. 4). Bredeson (2003) suggests that "metaphors are powerful cognitive and linguistic devices . . .

[with] suggestive comparisons" (p. 7). Patterns surface for your learners when you make design comparisons between two different items. In the next section, I compare the design process in architecture with the design process in education. As you read, remember that design is a dynamic thinking process. When constructivist theory is used as the fundamental way to design and construct daily lesson plans, you will have a better chance of involving your learners in an inquiry process. The intent is to give all students a chance to gain access to what you know while using their human senses and learning styles, not simply to learn what you know without thinking about it for themselves.

## Architectural Design

In this demonstration of metaphor as an instructional strategy, try to imagine yourself as an architect. You are asked to design a building to meet the needs of your client, who wants a home in the woods on a 5-acre parcel of land. Let's assume that your educational course work in architecture gave you background knowledge in how to design warehouses, skyscrapers, schools, malls, airports, houses, and other useful buildings. Specifically, you have the requisite background in physics, geometry, functions, and design, from which you will integrate essential knowledge and skills into a house design for your client.

Along with the course work you've taken, your own style preferences and personal background knowledge will inform the design. For example, your style preference includes Cape Cod houses, which originated in New England in the late 17th century. However, your personal background includes growing up in an established midwestern town, where you lived in a Victorian Gothic house with arches, pointed windows, and other artistic details borrowed from medieval cathedrals in Europe. In consultation with your client, you learn that he prefers a house style from 16th-century England known as an English Tudor. Together in a planning meeting, you begin to envision his home in the woods made of brick and timber, with high pinnacle gables, bay windows, and numerous chimneys. What you don't already know about the English Tudor style of design you will learn through interactions with your client, additional investigation and study, and trial and error.

Like teachers who do ongoing assessments of their learners, architects must serve the needs and interests of their clients in the design and delivery of the intended outcome. Any plan devoid of interactions between the designer and the client will result in a plan of futility. As in pedagogical design, architectural design requires ongoing research and development of the professional plan, leading to an increase in your personal practical knowledge (Connelly & Clandinin, 1988). Ubbes, Black, and Ausherman (1999) point out the following:

We especially need to emphasize the first step in educational planning in which the health needs and interests of learners are assessed initially and continually throughout the educational experience. This requires an assessment process of coming to know the learner from multiple perspectives, for instance, race, age, gender, intellectual, developmental, and many others. (p. 68)

Additional perspectives could come from class, culture, geographic location, and abilities.

Although it is possible to design something theoretically and not implement it or to design something and change it during the delivery, good design work seeks to solve a problem or meet a need. As the problem or need changes, the plan also changes to accommodate the preferences of your client, learners, or audience. There is a reason an architectural blueprint is drafted for consideration: A draft is often a preliminary plan, rough sketch, or written document. In teaching, lesson plans are often drafted and then revised many times to fit the changing educational milieu. We often use the term *refinement* when a design has gone through changes in form. Invariably, the design changes into a new form (or transforms) to meet the different needs of the learner or to solve new parts of the problem. The more we make design transparent to our learners, the better our chances of moving beyond the didactic habit of teaching as telling. Instead, the goal of constructivist teaching is to open up the space between the known and the unknown so that our learners are responsible for their own active constructions of meaning and can be encouraged to seek answers, both to their own questions and to fundamental questions of the disciplines.

## Change Orders Are Common

Change orders, or changes to the original order or plan, are common and necessary for customer satisfaction in the design and construction business. We experience this also in a restaurant when a person changes her order if the food arrives to the table in poor quality or the restaurant doesn't have the food as advertised in the menu. The customer suggests a change to her original order in consultation with the waitress or waiter. This analogous process is similar to what happens in a classroom when a teacher consults with a student who has unfinished or poor-quality work (but it also can result when an advanced student needs more challenging work to engage him in the learning task). In either educational situation, the lesson plan is adapted, refined, or extended to accommodate the needs and interests of one or many learners.

Planning with a focus on differentiating instruction for each student is very hard work that requires flexibility and changes to the original lesson plan. Once a novice teacher has gained time and experience with the basics of lesson design, she may be ready for this type of differentiated planning. In chapter 6, you will be prompted to accommodate differences by organizing your student assessments according to four different learning styles. If you have preference for a mastery learning style, you may require all students to complete certain lessons no matter what, even if some students have already mastered the health-related content or skills. You reason that practice is important for everyone. If you give students voice and choice in how they wish to meet the targeted learning outcomes, you are favoring a self-expressive learning style. When your students choose their own topics to investigate in depth, you are encouraging an understanding learning style. And when your students partner with one or more peers to investigate health-related concepts and skills, you are encouraging an interpersonal learning style.

In effective construction and design work, the design contractor and the client are in constant communication, usually prompted by the client, who exercises an active or passive role in the process. Job orders are customized to fit the customer's needs, interests, and preferences; client satisfaction is based on the original construction contract along with any change orders during the building process. Some homeowners place an order for their house with a contractor, then move in with their belongings as their first sign of involvement in the construction process. Rather than be active participants during the building process, they may exercise their rights to discuss specifications or make change requests after the move-in day. This is a form of reactionary living and learning rather than participatory living and learning.

In an educational context, a teacher who adopts a constructivist learning philosophy will often welcome and seek his learners' involvement during the design process. In more traditional educational settings, teachers design the lessons and then students are responsible for completing the activities or assignments. However, in more progressive educational settings, teachers and students are co-designers in the teaching–learning process. Such relational pedagogies help students "buy into" the learning task, encouraging them to be responsible for what they want to learn and to what extent they want to learn it in collaboration with others. Relational pedagogy is described more fully in chapter 7.

## Examples of Change Orders When Educating for Health

People, not work products, are the reasons health educators design and tailor health promotion and disease prevention messages. Although educational plans in the form of curricula or instructional units are designed to help different target populations, these plans are more effective when we first assess the interests, needs, and backgrounds of our learners, who vary by age, gender, racial ethnicity, culture, socioeconomic status, learning styles, and multiple intelligences.

Assessments are ongoing tools for determining what your learners know before, during, and after your educational intervention. As a novice teacher, you will be expected to target a classroom of children or youth with your health-related messages and skill-based lessons, but you will also need experience in tailoring key lessons for individual learners to ensure that learning takes place.

Writing and implementing change orders in health education take developmental experience and practice. For example, once you know how to educate for health in a particular content area (e.g., nutrition), you will gain expertise by modifying or refining your plans for a different target population. This might involve asking what your learners were taught in the preceding grade level or asking how well your learners mastered the concepts and skills at the next grade level after leaving your classroom. The inquiry process of design never ends.

Once you learn how to differentiate your plans for various age groups, you might focus on learners with a particular cultural tradition, language barrier, or special need. You can also learn how to adapt your plans by inviting speakers to your classroom or coordinating a lesson with a health-related organization in your school community. These examples emphasize how a health educator remains flexible in promoting health-related messages and educational lessons that meet the unique needs of various target populations, year after year. No matter how many learners of different backgrounds and motivations come under your influence, the concept of change will be a key factor in your educational design. In the last sentence, I deliberately chose the word *factor*. The fact that bears repeating is that change is a key factor in your educational design. You cannot teach the lesson the same way for a different group of learners. (Well, you could, but they may not learn it unless it is tailored and adapted to them.)

Teachers become effective instructional designers when they learn to use classroom assessment techniques (Angelo & Cross, 1993) to profile their learners. Teachers differ from architects or construction contractors, who look upon completed buildings as their end products. In education, the learner can be transformed by good curriculum or instructional design, but the person is not the final product in the design. Rather, people are central to the learning *process*. Although some teachers place themselves front and center in the classroom, this text encourages you to practice a student-centered model that places you on the side as a guide or facilitator for your students in their educational process. The end product becomes your learners' constructions of meaning (i.e., their learning or performances of understanding—not yours). In a constructivist educational design, both teachers and learners collaborate in the inquiry process to construct a new or different way to understand health-related concepts and skills. This collaborative process serves as a basis for classroom assessments and assignments so students gain new and different access to and practice with health-related information and skills.

# Role of Environment in Design

Now let's discuss how the environment plays an important role in an architectural plan. As the architect of an English Tudor home in the mountains of the southeastern United States, you will continue to make ongoing decisions about how to complete the project, drawing on the expertise of other professionals to coordinate the finishing touches of the design. Some environmental considerations might include how the building structure will interact with wind and weather patterns, how light will enter the house, and what views are possible through windows and doorways to the outside natural setting.

For the outside development of his home and property, your client will probably consult a landscape designer for guidance on plants, garden structures, and pond placement. For inside his home, your client may consult an interior designer for guidance on window treatments, furniture styles, and artistic decorations. As for the house design created by the architect, each decision by the landscape designer and the interior designer will be carefully made with the client for an overall effect. In schools, teachers, administrators, and other school professionals work together to improve the health and education status of children and youth. So much more care and concern should be considered for the learning environments in educational classrooms.

Effective designers, regardless of disciplinary background, will balance each element in their design with consideration of structure, function, and aesthetics. (You may wish to revisit figure 1.4 in chapter 1.) Although sight is often the most significant sense in architectural and landscape design, effective designers will also employ sound, smell, tactile texture, and taste to capture interest and imagination. When learning environments are structured to evoke the human senses in a safe and supportive way, students are able to function and learn more effectively, leading to a higher quality of life. A quality of life can be described as harmony in architectural and landscape design.

Harmony is described as a combination of individual elements leading to a pleasing or orderly whole. For example, your client can choose a visual effect of contrasting colors when painting the exterior of his Tudor-style home. He will need to select color combinations for the exterior of the house; for the windows and door trim; and for accent details such as shutters, doors, porch decks, and railings. The exterior of the house might be wood, natural masonry, stucco, or vinyl, depending on the client's preference for texture. When at least two elements of a project design are coordinated (e.g., color and texture of materials), the potential for harmony increases. Decisions for harmonious design should be planned for both outside and inside the home so that the unity of the individual elements results in pleasing patterns for the senses. Visual effects can come from natural plants and flowers and man-made art and sculptures. In the case of sound, rhythms of bird song, chirping crickets, water fountains, and stereo surround can be combined into harmonious effects.

## Establishing a Learning Environment

A learning environment helps you educate for health. Your students will need cooperative environments with a climate of acceptance and tolerance, not rejection and condemnation. By working together, you can establish an environment of empathy and concern versus an environment of selfishness and egocentrism (Deline, 1991).

A learning environment is skill based, conducted at an age-appropriate, child-centered pace, and allows time for practice. Teachers are responsible for moving learning into different environments as they educate for health. This means you must give your students time to practice the health-related skills outlined in the National Health Education Standards (Joint Committee on National Health Education Standards, 2007). If the environment is too busy and the curriculum too fast paced, kids will end up watching as the teacher demonstrates the skill and talks about it. A child-centered pace is compatible with the developmental need to learn in action, guided by the cues from teachers and caregivers. That is, when moving through the cafeteria line at school, the teacher cues students for effective decision making in action. Or while in game play at recess, the teacher cues students for conflict resolution strategies in specific contexts when needed. Or on the way to the restroom to wash hands, the teacher cues students for decision making on whether they also need water at the drinking fountain. These rehearsals in action are how patterns for health and wellness are established. Teachers can introduce the steps to skill development and give hypothetical situations to learn a skill, but students must step outside the structure of the curriculum to transfer and practice the skill in different places. Such migration of health-related skills into different places and situations increases the ability of children and youth to function as young adults.

## Principles of Pedagogy

Principles are a form of truth, though not always empirically based. They are often experienced with a pattern. Here are some pedagogical principles that make sense:

- Uncover and build on students' prior knowledge.
- Personalize information to make it more meaningful.
- Repeat and practice healthy patterns in new contexts.
- Engage the human senses to enhance capacity for information processing.
- Give time and space to learn habits of health and habits of mind.
- Design assignments so learners have access to what you know through an inquiry process.
- Educate for health using a variety of language elements, e.g., words, pictures, numbers, body language, rhythm, and environmental cues.
- Use transitions between lessons as opportunities to educate for health.

# Establish Conditions for Learning

Conditions for learning are learner-centered principles that are foundational to pedagogical design. For health-related information to be shared effectively, you must attend to, set up, or establish conditions "4" learning:

1. Developmentally appropriate—for different ages, intelligences, learning styles, and abilities (e.g., sensory-motor, cognitive-behavioral)
2. Culturally responsive—for different traditions, racial ethnicities, genders, and geographic locations
3. Body–brain compatible—for engaging the human senses, minimizing stress and threats, and increasing memory through information processing
4. Health enhancing—for practicing the habits of health and the habits of mind in an integrative pattern of life experiences

# What Is Developmentally Appropriate?

Developmental appropriateness is the first of four conditions for learning. Bunting (2004) writes about the transitional bridge between elementary children and middle school adolescents, citing that "much goes on in this brief developmental stretch—growth spurts, mood flights, fixations with appearance, worries about belonging, evolving freedoms, daunting responsibilities, unfolding talents and ambitions, giant steps toward empathy, and first fruits of womanhood and manhood" (p. 146).

This developmental period of puberty is highlighted by the changing sense of identity in early adolescence. By integrating educational, physiological, and psychological themes of well-being into the curriculum, youth are able to explore their sense of identity in different situations (Ubbes, 1999). Research findings on effective middle schools suggest that youth must be given positive social interaction with peers and adults; alternating periods of physical activity and adequate rest; structure and clear limits to ensure fairness and safety; and smaller subgroups or learning communities (Martin, 1993).

Adolescence is divided into three periods: early adolescence (ages 10-14), middle adolescence (ages 15-17), and late adolescence (ages 18 and up). Hillman (1991) claims that adolescence is "a continuous adaptation period with no clear boundaries between initiation into or exit from the period or its subperiods" (p. 4). He goes on to say that adolescence has a great variability and diversity, and "the enormous intra- and inter-individual behavioral variability is developmentally appropriate and represents both the charm and the challenge of working with this age group" (p. 4).

This text uses the human body as a metaphor for pedagogical design *and* as content for health promotion and wellness. In the former, the human body is analogous to a body of knowledge that you will need in educating for health. To understand the body of knowledge for health and wellness, you need to understand the knowledge structures of what students should know and be able to do in different contexts. These knowledge structures are like the human skeleton that gives the body and mind structure and protection for lifelong living and learning. In the latter, the human body and mind, with their 10 interdependent body systems, become the focus of the curriculum.

By designing health-promoting messages in the context of life and learning, we give people access to the signs, symbols, and patterns of wellness, not the symptoms of illness and disease. Young people do not need the disease-prevention messages of adults, who may have more motivations for studying the ill effects of high-risk behaviors. Teachers who teach predominantly about drugs, foods, and substances have misunderstood the health-promoting messages of wellness. What is needed in early and middle childhood curricula is a focus on the remarkable design of the body and mind through the hands-on, minds-on approach of habits of health and habits of mind, respectively. Habits of mind and habits of health are developmentally appropriate because they are concrete visuals for grades preK-8, narrowing the curriculum scope down to a manageable set of cognitive-behavioral abilities.

The school curriculum in health education must give students opportunities to be co-designers, not just consumers, of the lessons. Of course, teachers should teach and guide children through the health curriculum, but students also need space to explore their own inquiry-based projects beyond the curriculum. When students are given choices from which to select their own health topics to study, e.g., types of safety or types of beverages for hydration, they gain more understanding about their personal growth and development, which supports their identity formation.

For individuals to move from doing what they are told to doing what is personally advantageous, teachers must help children and youth analyze why they exercise and play; eat and drink nutritious foods; wash their hands; take safety precautions; nurture personal relationships; and get enough sleep, rest, and quiet time. When preteens begin shifting more to peer influences for some of their identity, there is often a period of time when they question or ignore parents, teachers, and caregivers in order to test their independent thinking. This period of independence still requires boundaries and guidelines set by grown-ups, but the determinants of health behaviors become multifactorial. That is, it is no longer as simple as "do this because I said so and do it as you've always done it."

Kids can be moved into healthful patterns of living by the helping hands of teachers, parents, and peers. You will learn how the habits of health and the habits of mind go hand in hand. You can learn to make a daily commitment in thoughts, words, and actions toward health and wellness. *Making* is an action word that implies taking an idea and putting it into action. We can say "make my day" when we want someone to do something we need. When we make a safety poster, we combine an idea with the use of our hands to make a product or prop that can be used to educate for health. When we write a script for a play, public service announcement, or health-promoting commercial, transforming our ideas into a message, we make a difference in the life of a young person who may need a cue to action for healthy decision making.

Too much information can be counterproductive, however. As adults, we need to be open and responsive to children and youth who have sensory overload. Kids who are overloaded in their body kinesthetic will tend to squirm and move around in their seats a lot or fuss with a tag in their clothing. Kids who are overloaded with too much heat or lighting may complain about headaches or breathing problems. Kids who are overstimulated by too much noise may be irritable or edgy. Kids who are understimulated by too little lighting may lack spontaneity and motivation to learn. You get the idea. Any host of environmental issues can either engage or interrupt the learning episode. There may be pleasure or pain. There may be focus or distractions. There may be benefits or barriers. You must be able to think with these mental schema so you can respond appropriately to each child.

The metaphor of sunlight can help us understand what to do with downcast faces and moody dispositions. The sun shines continuously on the earth, even when it is dark in the evening on your half of the world. The sun does not shine and go to sleep or shine when it feels like it. It shines continuously. Period. Scientists predict that our sun will not expire for about another 4 billion years (earth has existed for about 4.5 billion years), so we can assume that while we are teaching during the 21st century on this earth, the sun will continue to shine all the time. Children may think that the sun goes to sleep when they go to sleep, but the earth rotates away from the sun, leaving the area in darkness and the sun still shining. This light lives inside us and is kindled by joy.

So what can you make of this metaphor for teaching? You can use light and darkness to explain how people respond to life on earth. When educating for health, try to maintain your positive disposition even though your students may come and go with changing light and darkness. If you continue to be changed by your students' changing moods, very little teaching will be accomplished. This does not mean you ignore all negative emotions and acknowledge all positive emotions. You are wise to acknowledge people's emotions by making observations of facts: It sounds like . . . or it looks like . . . or it feels like. . . . "I" statements are probably least effective when you are interacting with a sad or moody person. Instead, sentences that begin with "it" help establish an objective and neutral position. This also gives you the ability to shine light on the situation without joining in the other person's mood.

The greatest gift we can give ourselves and others is to remain enlightened by the exchange and not be extinguished by the darkness. Empathetic teachers can see the mask of the other without wearing the mask. Many of our interactions with people are simply trial and error. Even family members who have lived with each other for long periods of time cannot predict the thoughts, feelings, and actions of their loved ones with high accuracy, nor should they be expected to "know" and "act" in a certain way. Life is best lived in a 24-hour period of time and renewed each day. Although we can anticipate some people's patterns, especially closer friends and family members, we cannot do so with success if we are expecting them to respond based only on our needs and points of view. Wellness gives us an opportunity to renew ourselves each day, and conversations should be renewed as well.

Children and youth who live through major challenges and disasters become wise through their experiences. We must give young people access to their wisdom by promoting nonverbal environments for sharing what they know through the visual and performing arts. Not all kids are able to express themselves through words. Pictures, numbers, body language, and rhythms are also important ways to show what they know and feel about a topic, issue, or problem.

When disasters of weather, war, accidents, or the unexpected threaten the human population, darkness seems to come and linger over us like a black cloud. In time, a few bright smiles shine light in the shadows to help other people gain access to their thoughts and feelings. We all can move through these changing moments to another point of view. In teaching, we can plan for these metamorphoses, but the best ones often take us by surprise. Loren Eiseley, former director of the Newport Aquarium in Covington, Kentucky, says, "If there is magic on this planet, it is contained in water. . . . Its substance reaches everywhere; it touches the past and prepares the future." When light enters water, it refracts and bends. It can be broken into the different colors of the spectrum to form a rainbow. So as we change our position to see the light in a new form, we are reminded of the hope of a new day and our next moment of transformation.

## What Is Culturally Sensitive?

Cultural sensitivity is the second of four conditions for learning. *Healthy People 2010* (U.S. Department of Health and Human Services, 2000) acknowledges the barrier of cultural disparities in educating all people for health. Issues of equity remain integral to education, health, and communication contexts because, as Stoy (2000) argues, legitimate differences exist among ethnic, cultural, and gender groups, calling for health educators to develop an action plan for intercultural competence. Professional preparation programs can use the lens of communication and language patterns to advance health education. For example, an anthropologist, Geertz (1973), defines culture as "a historically transmitted pattern of meaning embodied in symbols, a system of inherited conceptions expressed in symbolic form by means of which men communicate, perpetuate, and develop their knowledge about and attitudes toward life" (p. 16). Hall (1976) points out that individual members of a community can have a common understanding of symbols and representations for communication but vary greatly in thoughts, feelings, and behaviors. Such perspectives on culture and intercultural competence must be an important component of professional preparation in health education, because culture influences our identity formation, our communication patterns, and how we learn (Stoy, 2000).

Before we can appreciate and honor the cultural diversity that exists in the world, we need to be able to honor our own dignity and worth. This section shows three tables in which the results are damaging to the individual. Our severe judgments of self and others can have a devastating effect on our health and well-being. In tables 3.2 and 3.3, we find examples of dysfunctional thinking. In both cases, our intellectual health is faulty and needs some guidance from helpful friends, family members, and colleagues. Unfortunately, middle school youth often fall prey to this faulty thinking. In table 3.4, we see three different behavioral patterns that are used when communicating. Although the goal is to demonstrate assertive behavior as much as possible in our lives, there are times when we display aggressive and passive behaviors. In many cases, the predominant use of dysfunctional behaviors that emerge from aggressive and passive responses is harmful to self and others. When educating for health, it is important to teach young people what dysfunctional thinking and actions look like, sound like, and feel like. We can all learn to design our thinking and actions to be more culturally sensitive so we can boost our core identities that are in formation.

### Table 3.2   Automatic Negative Thinking (ANT) That Compromises Our Cognitive-Emotional Identities

| ANT | Description of that ANT |
| --- | --- |
| All or nothing thinking | Thoughts are all good or all bad |
| "Always" thinking | Thinking in words such as *always, never, no one, everyone, every time, everything* |
| Focusing on the negative | Able to see only the bad in a situation |
| Fortune telling | Predicting the worst possible outcome to a situation |
| Mind reading | Believing you know what another person is thinking even though he or she hasn't told you |
| Thinking with your feelings | Believing negative feelings without questioning them |
| Guilt beatings | Thinking in words such as *should, must, ought, have to* |
| Labeling | Attaching a negative label to yourself or to someone else |
| Blame | Blaming someone else for the problems you have |

## Table 3.3   Cognitive-Emotional Bugs

| Type of Cognitive-Emotional Bug | Description of Cognitive-Emotional Bug |
|---|---|
| Mind reader bug | The mind reader bug convinces its victims that we read and anticipate the thoughts and feelings of others. |
| Blame bug | The blame bug tells us it's much easier to blame someone else instead of accepting responsibility in a situation. |
| Invalidator bug | This gloomy little insect uses every opportunity to cast a negative shadow on positive events. |
| Perfection bug | The perfection bug tricks us into setting unattainable goals and then pounces on us with shame and humiliation when we fail to meet them. |
| Past bug | The past bug freezes its victims in a false world of *might have beens* instead of facing the present realities of life. |
| Future bug | The future bug saps our energy by encouraging us to worry about an imaginary future, leaving us little strength to face the real world. |
| Should bug | As long as the should bug keeps us in a fantasy mentality and away from reality, we will be stuck in a world of demands and condemnation. |
| Magnifier bug | Using global words such as *always*, *never*, *everybody*, and *nobody* may be a sign that we are being influenced by this bug. |

Permission granted by Equipping Ministries Int'l, Cincinnati, OH. EMIGROW@equipmin.org.

## Table 3.4   Communication Styles: Aggressive, Passive, and Assertive

| | Aggressive | Passive | Assertive |
|---|---|---|---|
| **Definition** | Leaves out others' rights, feelings, and needs. Acts against others by getting what he or she wants by dominating, manipulating, and humiliating others. | Leaves self out by not expressing needs or feelings or by denying or letting others violate his or her rights. | Speaks up for self appropriately while considering the needs, wishes, and rights of others. Practices open, honest, two-way communication. |

|  | Aggressive | Passive | Assertive |
|---|---|---|---|
| **Why used?** | To reach immediate goals; to express anger | To avoid unpleasantness or conflict | To communicate effectively; to feel good about self; to get needs met |
| **Results** | Accomplishes short-term goals but alienates others; ends up lonely and bitter | Needs aren't met; feels frustrated and disappointed; has low self-esteem | May not reach short-range goals; may compromise or go for alternatives; usually reaches long-term goals; has healthy relationships; feels good about self for being open and honest with others |
| **Verbal cues** | Blames or accuses others; uses sarcasm; displays an air of superiority | Rambles; beats around the bush; overapologizes; does not say what he or she really thinks; has a weak or unsteady voice or no response at all | Clearly, directly, and honestly states feelings; uses "I" messages |
| **Nonverbal cues** | Makes shows of strength; has a loud or brittle voice; has a cold, detached look; assumes a rigid or haughty posture; uses jerky, dominating gestures such as finger pointing or table pounding; intrudes into others' space | Assumes a slouched posture; has downcast, averted, or tearful eyes; has sticky or cold hands; uses nervous gestures | Listens well to others; assumes an upright posture; speaks in a relaxed, well-modulated voice; maintains good eye contact |

# What Is Body–Brain Compatible?

Body-brain compatibility is the third of four conditions for learning. Our sense organs (ears, eyes, nose, tongue, skin, and proprioceptors) transmit outside sensory information to the brain as neurochemical and neuromechanical messages. These sensory messages are then interpreted by the brain to make it possible for us to hear, see, smell, taste, or touch. Without the brain, we would not be able to perceive, respond, or attend to the world's messages.

We often process sensory-motor and cognitive cues simultaneously. Recent research shows that the amygdala perceives threatening or stressful situations in a preferential way before the prefrontal cortex has a chance to think. This is called an emotional hijacking, because our neurochemical response preempts our thoughtful responses from the prefrontal cortex, which serves as the "pilot" control center of the brain. The brain processes sensory and motor information side by side in the sensory cortex and motor cortex, respectively, which activates affective sensory or efferent motor pathways to the body. Your prefrontal cortex in the area of your forehead gives you executive control over your behaviors. However, your prefrontal "thinking" cortex does not fully develop until you are in your mid- to late 20s.

We can consciously focus our attention on what we want to see or hear or touch, but some of our responses to the world are not attended to by our conscious minds. A great deal of information processing occurs automatically through the autonomic nervous system. For example, you do not need to consciously attend to the medulla oblongata in your brain stem, which controls (with other body organs and its neurotransmitters or hormones) your respiration. You can consciously attend to your breathing when learning to swim or when playing a musical instrument, but a great deal of practice is needed to teach your nervous system, especially your conscious brain and sensory-motor neuronal pathways, to control your breathing pattern of intensity and frequency. Once your neuronal networks have sufficiently rehearsed this conscious request, your nervous system and its interconnected neuronal pathways can go into autopilot (referred to as automatic memory) when you call on them in the future. But you still need to initiate the movement with conscious thought.

Of course, there are exceptions to automatic conscious thoughts. Our bodies have a masterful built-in reflex system that removes our hands from hot objects or refuses to eat something that smells spoiled. Our bodies are remarkably complex, with the ability to react reflexively under both unconscious and conscious thought. For example, some people can anticipate a fly ball coming toward them, and others may not be as expert. Your sensory-motor coordination requires prior knowledge to tell your brain how to respond. Your human senses process sensory information from the environment all the time except during sleep. In the case of the fly ball, your eyes must be able to see the ball, then your muscles coordinate your arm and leg movements, while your ears help you keep your balance during the catch. This sensory-motor coordination becomes natural with practice; much of it is conscious, and yet some of it is unconscious to your mind.

Your brain and body are still working on your behalf even if you don't focus or attend to them. In the case of moving toward a ball to catch it, your eyes, ears, and limbs must integrate their visual, auditory (balance), and kinesthetic perceptions to coordinate the movement. This sensory integration is remarkably patterned with practice and repetition. It works a little awkwardly at first, until your senses and your thinking (and reflexive) nervous system coordinate the reading of visual, auditory, and kinesthetic cues from the environment, but patterns are eventually established for this movement. Your frontal cortex (cognitive thinking brain that makes decisions from sensory cues in the environment) will coordinate with the cerebellum at the back of your brain to make these sensory-motor patterns more efficient and natural. If you spend time practicing this sensory-motor skill, you will be able to catch balls of various colors, shapes, and sizes under different conditions (e.g., on the run, in the rain, with sun glare, with or without special hand coverings). These contextual changes in catching a ball speak to your growing expertise and sophistication in learning. Whether it involves brushing your teeth, washing your hands, or another motor skill, you will need to understand the importance of body–brain compatibility when educating for health.

## What Is Health Enhancing?

Health enhancement is the fourth condition for learning. Preventive medicine—which uses the operative word *preventive* to describe its intention—occurs at three levels: primary, secondary, and tertiary. Primary prevention is also called health promotion. Health promotion begins with people who are basically healthy and seeks a development of community and individual measures to help them develop lifestyles that can maintain and enhance their state of well-being. It is through primary prevention that we can educate for health, although secondary and tertiary prevention also use education to help people seek health-related screenings and health-enhancing rehabilitation, respectively.

In health promotion, the concept of wellness is used "to express the quality of living each day" (Bonaguro, 1981, p. 502). The goal of wellness is to help people manage their perceptions of everyday living. When we talk about a quality of living, we are referring to a very subjective concept that encompasses one's satisfaction and happiness with daily experiences. For that reason, wellness may not often be used as an objective measure for research purposes in health education. However, wellness can help individuals think about their daily habits of health and habits of mind.

The reality of living in a democracy where we can celebrate voice and choice is a hardship for some individuals who have limited access to knowledge, education, and health care. As a young professional, you must be taught about the marginalization of certain people and professions from different points of view so you will know what to look for, including how to understand and negotiate regulation and legislation of education and health policies. The sooner you learn to grapple with top-down, hierarchical structures and to participate in opportunities for shared decision making, the richer your professional growth and development will be.

## Thinking as a Health Promoter

In certain disciplines, experts are encouraged to think like historians, artists, mathematicians, or scientists. In this text, you are encouraged to think like a health promoter who educates for health. In order to think like a health promoter, you will need adequate background knowledge in personal health and in the principles and pedagogy of health education. Finding the time to learn new health content in a skill-based health curriculum in the middle of a busy teaching week can be challenging. Although professionals could argue that student connections can be found in all academic subjects, a wise teacher will respect the necessary time needed for skill development in health education—because the student *is* the curriculum. No other school subject, except physical education, has a curriculum of human beings. Sure, you will study about humans creating art, making music, solving equations, and making scientific discoveries, but health education places the human being central to the curriculum of life.

Health education uses the thinking of other subject matter to explore human life. For example, when we think like scientists, we explore the mysteries of sound and light as changing energy forms. In health education, we explore how we perceive sound and light through our senses and how to promote the health and well-being of ourselves and others. When we think like mathematicians, we explore the numerical patterns of sound and wave frequencies as algorithms or physics. In health education, we explore how sound protection and light protection increase our personal health, with an emphasis on our ears, eyes, and skin through important hygiene and safety actions.

When we think like historians, we use the basic questions from history to guide our curriculum work in health education. When a daily newspaper or news broadcast is released each morning and throughout the day, the reporter answers the historical questions of "what, where, when, why, and who or with whom?" Reporters may also go deeper to uncover the "how" and "to what extent" questions of the situation. We can then translate the same questions into health actions. What exercise did you do or food did you eat today? Where and when did you do this health action? Why did you choose that particular exercise or food? With whom did you exercise or eat? How do you feel now? And to what extent did that contribute to your overall wellness today? These questions form the story of health.

The word *story* evolved from the word *history*. Williams (2003) suggests the following:

> The historian seeks to discover order and structure in the chaos and messiness of the past. The historian also *constructs* order and structure by creating a narrative or an argument, based on verifiable evidence. Historians know they live in a present where bias and interpretation of the past abound. They understand their own bias. Yet they try to be objective. In addition to telling a story, *they develop a persuasive argument* on the basis of the evidence, an argument that they believe is reasonable and accurate. They write about context, as well as text. They identify causes that will help explain how or why events happened the way they did. They seek *understanding* and *empathy* with individuals in another time and place. (p. 12)

How will these same questions work if you are focused on children and youth from a social health perspective? Teachers are often adept at using these questions when dealing with misbehaving children or personal conflicts. However, teachers must eventually learn to deal with student interactions as their first curriculum (i.e., their modus operandi) and not their last. In health education, you will focus on building and enhancing relationships that promote health. These include students' relationships with the information, with the teacher, with their peers, and with the home, school, and community. In the next sections of this chapter, we explore the historical, social, and linguistic context of educating for health, which may help you frame your philosophy.

# Historical Significance of Knowledge Construction

The first human language emerged roughly 150,000 years ago in East Africa, while written forms of language date back approximately 6,000 years (Dreifus, 2001). At present, 5,000 languages are spoken in the world. Societies come to understand language through oral and written histories, genealogies, folk tales, and books of different genres—from narrative picture books to expository informational texts.

During the Middle Ages in Europe, the church ruled religious thought and all scientific thought. The period of the Enlightenment, which coexisted with the Renaissance in the arts and the Reformation in religion, was marked by the spread of knowledge outside the church to the general population. Before the 1500s, only clerics knew how to read because they were the only ones who were educated. Church services were held in Latin to "separate" church leaders from the masses, and the general population was not allowed to read sacred texts so that their interpretation could be controlled. By keeping knowledge within the authority of a few, the church could remain in the superior position of interpreter of information.

During the 1500s, it was against the law to translate sacred texts into the common languages of the people (e.g., French, German, and English). This continued to give church leaders the sole authority to interpret the Bible, the sacred text of the Christian church. For centuries, access to church doctrine was possible only for those who knew the language.

During the entire Middle Ages, Latin served as an international means of communication, with virtually all the communications of the church, governments, and schools expressed in Latin (Wallbank, Taylor, & Bailkey, 1975). A rise in literature of the vernacular (common language) began to appear in the 12th century, led by Dante in Italy and Chaucer in England. Chaucer wrote his novel *The Canterbury Tales* in Middle English circa 1387, providing popular literature that people wanted to read and giving rise to increased interest in literacy. In essence, people were motivated to learn to read because there was something "novel" and worthwhile to read and because the story was being talked about on the streets and in neighborhoods. Whereas early English was influenced by the Germanic language of Anglo-Saxon, Middle English surfaced from the dialect of Oxford, England.

John Wycliff, a contemporary of Chaucer, wrote other popular works that people wanted to read, helping to give rise to the Enlightenment period, which started the spread of literacy—and with it shared knowledge and enlightened thought. Wycliff, a professor at Oxford (England), prepared an English translation of the Bible. Writings by Calvin and Zwingli in Switzerland 200 years later added to this literacy momentum and to the spirit of individual freedom in revolt against medieval authority. With the invention of movable type in 1450, printed material became much cheaper and widely available. People began to shift from an oral tradition of storytelling to writing.

The earliest universities grew from unorganized groups of scholars and students in Bologna, Italy, and Paris, France, mostly stimulated by Greek and Arabic knowledge from previous centuries. Some achievements of the early Greek tradition were democratic governments elected by the people; great architecture; and the notable philosophies of Socrates, Plato, and Aristotle. Achievements from the ancient Middle East include invention of the wheel, the study of astronomy, establishment of the 24-hour day, and creation of alphabets from picture drawings known as hieroglyphics and cuneiform. Before these Greek and Arab accomplishments were made, achievements in China included the invention of paper, the invention of gunpowder, and the invention of acupuncture to treat illnesses. During the rule of the Han (202 BC), the Chinese also studied astronomy and engineering.

Some scholars suggest that the start of the Reformation in religious thought can be attributed to German reformer Martin Luther, who posted his Ninety-Five Theses on the door of a parish church in protest against the church. The posting of information on a church door in the 1500s is the equivalent of posting something on the Internet today so that others can read it. Luther was frustrated with the narrow interpretation of authority, including how that authority abused its power over the people. This action sparked a ripple effect of others who protested the authority of the church, foreshadowing the Protestant movement that followed almost two centuries later into America. In Western thought today, religious beliefs vary by denominations or forms of Protestantism. This proliferation of multiple forms of Protestantism ranks third to other major religions in the world (e.g., Buddhism, Confucianism, Hinduism, Islam, Judaism, Eastern Orthodox, Roman Catholicism, Shinto, and Taoism, among many others) (*NY Public Library Desk Reference,* 1989).

As people began to realize that knowledge could be gained through scientific investigation and systematic thought, the church began to lose its place of power. When the institution of the church was in charge, people were forced to believe the doctrines and teachings of the church as being in authority, even though the Bible warns against such justifications. Those scientists who gave an alternative point of view regarding the position of the stars, sun, and planets, such as Kepler and Galileo, were imprisoned for their ideas. Unfortunately, this set up a tendency for dichotomous thinking, in that people had to have faith alone or risk losing their lives for their scientific interpretation of how things worked.

The Enlightenment period also marked the spread of knowledge outside the church to the general population by increasing their access to knowledge. By today's standards, we have come a long way, because many educated people of all disciplinary backgrounds do integrate the shared values of faith and reason. Instead of using "either/or" thinking to determine what is acceptable and what is not acceptable, people can hold faith and reason simultaneously as expressed by "and/both" thinking. This is important for teachers and educators to understand.

By literal definition, information can be explained as being "in formation," leading to many forms of interpretation. Many educational scholars have written about the moral dimensions of teaching, even though many teachers still fear that they cannot talk about religion and the church or don't know how to walk the fine line between religion and faith. Although this book is not the place for this type of discussion, it is important to posit the role of the church in limiting access to knowledge and educating the masses in its earliest history.

Today, the institution of the church is a favored setting for different health education programs. Educating for health in faith-based institutions, including hospitals that are affiliated with different churches, can be found in the form of healthy heart campaigns, lupus awareness programs, and five-a-day fruit and vegetable initiatives, to name a few. In addition, parish health ministries run the gamut from blood pressure screenings to cancer prevention screenings with their parishioners. These programs are found throughout faith-based institutions, family and social service agencies, community organizations, and workplaces. What is important is that we respect and honor how people choose to live their lives and find ways to educate for health where they work and play. For example, some of the greatest health disparities in the United States are among African Americans and Hispanics, for whom parish health ministries are able to give greater access to health information and screenings.

## A Story of Professional Integration

The Renaissance era gave rise to many different artists, musicians, and writers who expressed their views and ideas more and more freely, leading to incredible growth and diversity in aesthetic works during this time. Imagine meeting an artist today who is valued as a master of three artistic genres: painting, sculpture, and architecture. By today's standards, an artist may be gifted in one of these artistic media. But that was not the case for Michelangelo, who is judged by many to be the greatest among other Italian artists (e.g., Giotto, Donatello, Botticelli, da Vinci) because of his multiple aesthetic representations.

Michelangelo, known famously by only his first name, was born in the Republic of Florence in the very heart of the Renaissance—a time of rebirth between the 14th and 16th centuries. Stanley (2000) summarizes this period:

> Though the Renaissance spread all over Europe, it was born in Italy, where magnificent Roman ruins were constantly being unearthed in fields and vineyards and at construction sites. The discovery of those ancient buildings, as well as masterpieces of antique sculpture and Greek and Roman writings on science and philosophy, inspired a whole new way of thinking and a whole new kind of art. (p. 11)

This account is important because it teaches us that great works are often built upon a historical context and are inspired from the past and present experiences of the master in the midst of his (or her) contemporaries, who have their own interpretations and perspectives of the time.

About the same time that fellow Italian Christopher Columbus set sail from Spain to find a New World, Michelangelo began to travel from Florence to Venice to Bologna to Rome in his early to mid-20s to work as an artist. Michelangelo sculpted his famous work the *Pieta* in Rome, his *David* in Florence, and later the paintings on the ceiling of the Sistine Chapel in Rome. He accomplished other remarkable pieces, including being an architect of St. Peter's Cathedral in 1547 at the age of 70. During his last 17 years of life, Michelangelo donated his time and refused to accept any payment, saying he did it for the "good of his soul" (Stanley, 2000, p. 45). At the age of 89, Michelangelo spoke of how much he regretted "dying just as I am beginning to learn the alphabet of my profession" (p. 48).

So what does this have to do with educating for health using a constructivist approach? Early in this book, I suggested that your personal and professional lives will become integrated over the course of your career. The degree of integration will require you to come to know your personal lifestyle and professional work style in the context of your changing needs and interests. You might think about how you will be influenced by people, places, and events in your life. Like Michelangelo, you will be shaped by your genetics, experiences, education, geography, and time in history. To fulfill his life's work, Michelangelo had to continually seek financial support through patrons who commissioned his aesthetic works of sculpture, paintings, and architecture. Although you will not need to raise money for your work directly, you may end up spending some of your own money in order to meet your needs and interests when educating for health.

You will also need to find support for your ideas from administration and parents, including people outside your immediate influence. When you choose to transport your ideas into different spheres of influence that require movement and travel from one place to another, you will have a larger impact on the world. Some of your colleagues may grow their spheres of influence on a local level first and expand to more global levels. Or some of your colleagues may start at the macrolevel and move into smaller influences at different times. In the end, educators are all responsible for interpreting knowledge and transforming information into multiple ways of knowing to be accessed by many different users. When we educate for health, we give people direction in how to be health literate, especially how to access and use information and services in ways that are health enhancing.

## Developing a Philosophy to Educate for Health

When you begin to educate for health, you might take inspiration from historical and contemporary works (e.g., books, art, music, film, speeches, architecture). As you continue to refine your understanding of the unique gifts and talents you offer as an educator, you will also learn to build on other people's ideas and give them credit for the ways they have helped shape your teaching philosophy. You might envision your educational platform as a place where you take people from where they are now to where they want to be, including where you want them to be.

One of your most difficult challenges may be uncovering your philosophy with regard to positions of power in your classroom. Who owns knowledge? Who should decide or legislate what you should know and be able to do as a teacher? Do you agree or disagree with educational standards that frame what students should know and be able to do in eight different subjects?

Armstrong (2003) highlights some key questions about the use of different books for understanding both personal and social perspectives:

> How does this text speak or not speak to you personally? How does it reflect or not reflect your social world? How does it raise questions for you about the ways in which people of a different race, gender, ethnic group, religion, or sexual orientation live? . . . How do these texts mirror (or not mirror) the racial, ethnic, gender, religious, and sexual preference identifications of the students? (p. 105)

In the picture book *Let's Talk About Race*, Julius Lester (2005) introduces the concept of race as only one component of a person's story. The book opens with these words: "I am a story. So are you. So is everyone." Later, the reader is asked to do the following:

> Suppose, just suppose, one day we—I mean everyone in the whole world—decided to take off all our clothes and all our skin and all our hair. Then we would do what we do normally every day—go to school, go to work, play and shop. Everything would be normal except we would look at each other and couldn't tell who was a man, who was a woman, who was white, black, Hispanic or Asian. . . . Which story shall we believe? The one that says "My race is better than yours?" Or the one we just discovered for ourselves: Beneath our skin I look like you and you look like me. (pp. 18-19)

This story highlights important social lessons, with a small bias on biological differences between genders, but there are significant truths to explore: that we are more alike than different. Or as bell hooks (2004) says so poignantly in *Skin Again*,

The skin I'm in is just a covering. It cannot tell my story. The skin I'm in is just a covering. If you want to know who I am you have got to come inside and open your heart way wide. The skin I'm in looks good to me. It will let you know one small way to trace my identity. (p. 16)

Armstrong (2003) states, "Nobody invents a language, creates a book, coins a word, or utters a meaningful sentence as a single individual operating within a cultural vacuum. All of this linguistic activity takes place within a rich social milieu" (pp. 98-99). He offers the following examples of how literacy is often associated with power:

An 8-year-old writes the words "Go Away!" on a piece of paper and tacks it to his bedroom door, and suddenly he shapes the social world around him in a tangible way that powerfully expresses the temporary distance he wishes to have with respect to that world. A 6th grader writes an essay on environmental waste that helps to create a recycling program for her school. A teenager writes a passionate love letter to a girl he just met and discovers to his joy that it serves to transform an accidental meeting into a significant romantic relationship. An adult writes an article for a local newspaper on recent layoffs in his community and generates a political action group from among several of its unemployed readers. (p. 99)

Armstrong continues:

Students need to learn that there are many different kinds of texts, and that each text is uniquely embedded in a societal context. There is text in library books, text on television, text in high-stakes tests, text on the blackboard, text on a cafeteria menu. And each of these texts differs in their social purposes and aims. (p. 99)

## Design and Style

In matters of taste, style, life, relationships, and faith, we have important distinctions to make. We must learn to honor what is unique about self, but we may wander onto a slippery slope if we allow self to matter more than the contributions we make to society.

We can discern our paths of individuality, but our work and play need to be reflected through our relationships. We can put our whole minds into our work and be successful. But we must also know how to negotiate our ideas with the public and launch with care. When our work does not meet the inclusive standard of society, we can separate ourselves from others in arrogance, judgment, or ridicule, but that sets a foundation for elitism that cuts us from needed support. Instead, we may choose to integrate ourselves with society, which sets the foundation for educating for health.

## Role of Literacy in Educating for Health

Young children need to understand the function of print and how it works. For example, books written in English are read from front to back, and the print on the page is made up of words. Words are composed of letters and are separated by spaces (concept of *word*). The print, which is speech that is written down, carries meaning (concept of *print*). To make sense of print, children need to understand its directionality of front to back, top to bottom, and beginning to end. The words are composed of letters with distinct shapes that when grouped together form words with specific names (concept of *letter*). Teachers, parents, and caregivers help children learn these concepts through repeated exposures to books, environmental print, and oral language. In print-rich environments, children observe adults choosing from a menu, stopping a vehicle at a stop sign, and selecting products at the supermarket (Strickland & Schickedanz, 2004). Each of these examples is a way to educate for health.

Strickland and Schickedanz (2004) place children into different organizational patterns in the classroom: whole group, small group, and individualized one-on-one sessions. These instructional groupings are a form of differentiated instruction, and when coupled with scaffolding, the learner has a better chance of succeeding at a task. The scaffolding process begins when an adult controls the learning by demonstrating or modeling a skill. In step 2, the adult guides the learning by inviting the student to try the task. In the third step of the scaffolding process, the adult monitors the learning by inviting the student to try the skill on her own and helping her when needed. In the example of scaffolding for reading, the teacher reads aloud, and then children read along, followed by children reading alone.

In a health-related example, children learn how to set a goal for getting enough sleep. The parents and teacher help to monitor this habit of health by posting charts at home and in the classroom. By using the charts the children can keep track of their consistent practice of getting adequate sleep. It may also be a good time to track the number of books or pages read each night, since literacy is a critical skill for health.

Phonemic awareness is the ability to hear, identify, and manipulate the individual sounds (phonemes) in spoken words. Strickland and Schickedanz (2004) note that physical growth and development include gross motor development (e.g., large muscle movement), fine motor development (e.g., small muscle movement of fingers and hands), and sensory-perceptual development (e.g., receipt, recognition, and interpretation of information that comes through the senses).

## Objective Knowing and Subjective Knowing

Some professionals express worry or raise objections when we speak about constructivism as a theory for teaching and learning. There are reasons for these objections. Since I wish to encourage you to use constructivist theory when educating for health, it may be useful to compare and contrast subjective thinking and objective thinking. These terms were used in the last chapter when describing learning styles, so there is good reason to cover them in more detail here.

*Subjective* is an adjective that describes your feelings or opinions rather than actual facts. Because subjective thoughts exist in your mind, or in the thoughts and feelings of the speaker, writer, teacher, or painter, there is little external control or understanding about what is going on in your head or, more explicitly, in your patterned neuronal responses to a stimulus. To study subjective thought, we must change the adjective into other forms of speech so that *subjective* becomes either a noun (e.g., subject: an area, a person, or a thing that is being studied) or a verb (e.g., subject: to force to endure).

You study different subjects all the time in your academic life. You can refer to the academic disciplines as subjects (e.g., health education, social studies, mathematics), and you can also study subjects within the disciplines that can be both topical (i.e., more specific) or conceptual (i.e., more abstract). Therefore, teachers who know a subject well are often interested in your knowing the subject just as well as they do. The truly interesting fact about the verb form of *subject* is that often teachers can subject their students to a great deal of rigor in order for them to learn a subject. When professionals subject their students to reasonable, but sometimes unreasonable, demands that may or may not fit their developmental readiness, the hierarchy of the expert and the novice are realized.

In social studies, we see example after example of how people exert their need for power, control, and recognition through hierarchical levels of political standing. In health care, we see examples of how poverty unreasonably determines whether individuals, and even groups of people by culture or social standing, have limited or no access to health care. In education, we also have examples of educators at different levels determining the entire curriculum for what students will know and do without any input or choice from students. This statement supports the need for constructivist theory in education (and in life) so we can do as Palmer (1998) suggests by designing pedagogy that honors the "little" stories of students *and* the "big" stories of the disciplines and traditions; that honors the voice of the individual *and* the voice of the group; that honors and supports solitude *and* surrounds solitude with community.

Have you begun to realize why subjectivism is an important side of the educational story? Let's look at subjective thought in educating for health. Your subjective self cannot be controlled or understood by other people because we cannot access your thoughts and feelings unless we ask you to disclose your subjective notions or you do it of your own free will. In education, the higher we go and the more sophisticated we become in our intellectual lives, the more the intellect tends to overshadow and sometimes even ignore or silence the emotions and motivations of others. In contrast, in early childhood education, children come into your classrooms with many emotions exposed and sometimes hidden, and in middle childhood education, youth are often recognized by their emotive changing identities. So then, where does subjective thinking fit within a developmental model of education?

Constructivist teaching and learning are important when educating for health because we need to help our learners get access to valid and reliable health information and services from which they can construct their personal meaning for health and well-being. Students still need a designated place and time in the academic curriculum to personalize their learning and explore how to live a quality of life. Health education is a discipline in which the human being matters as the subject of study. This is built on the rationale that health is foundational to learning. Without health, one cannot learn. Without wellness, one cannot learn well.

Richard Paul, a noted educational philosopher, helps educators know how to think about subject matter with a distinction between facts, opinions, and evidence. In Paul's three-part thinking model (1999), facts are named as a single system of thought. We can ask questions with one right answer and expect children and youth to respond with a statement that can be proven true. For example, a health-related question with one right answer is "What is the name of the human sense that uses your eyes to see?" The answer is sight. We can also ask questions in which there can be as many answers as there are different people or human preferences. This category of thinking is known as opinions. We often ask questions of opinion when we want to know a person's preferences or needs. For example, an opinion question in health education is "Is it easy or hard for you to eat breakfast every day?"

And finally, when we ask questions that require evidence and reasoning within multiple systems of thought (or disciplines), we ask students to make a factual case by citing their sources of knowledge and to reason why and to what extent these facts support the evidence. For example, an evidence-based question in health education is "Can you

demonstrate three ways to refuse tobacco when offered ᴀ
a real-life context, if the cigarette is refused and the targᴇ
is to refuse, then you can go on to make judgments as to whᵢ
the three refusal strategies was more effective than the otheɪ
also ask students to find evidence why tobacco use is the nuᵢ        ᴊe
preventable cause of death in this country. You can build a case wᵢ,ₙ one,
two, three facts, and more, supporting the claim that tobacco products
should not be used by anyone.

This is where subjective norms play a role in health education, because
a person can be subjected to a variety of situational and environmental
cues in a specific context for accepting or rejecting a cigarette. We can
target our health-related messages for what to do when a cigarette is
offered to groups of preteens, but we may need to investigate the subtle
and real contextual cues present for each person. By definition, a subjective norm is "the individual's belief of whether or not people who
are important to the individual approve or disapprove of the behavior,
combined with the individual's motivation to comply with the expectations of those people" (McMillan & Connor, 2003, p. 321). This line
of reasoning takes us to several health education theories, such as the
Theory of Reasoned Action developed by Fishbein (Gillmore et al., 2002),
in which health behavior is examined through behavioral intentions and
decision making via intrapersonal and interpersonal factors; the Theory
of Planned Behavior developed by Ajzen (Montano & Kasprzyk, 2002),
which builds upon the Theory of Reasoned Action with the addition
of the construct of perceived behavioral control based on past experiences; and the Transtheoretical Model of Behavior Change (Prochaska &
DiClemente, 1983; Walton et al., 1999), which assesses readiness to be
healthy or stay healthy along a continuum of five stages of change. Subjective norms may also play an important role in differentiating between
targeted and tailored public health messages for specific populations or
groups of people (Kreuter & Wray, 2003).

## Role of Neuroscience in Constructivist Theory: Zone of Proximal Development

Interneurons communicate when there is an action potential. Learning
occurs when a neurochemical process triggers the release of a neurotrans-
mitter at the synaptic gap between two neurons. We can also have gaps
in our learning when we do not make an extra effort to connect what we
are learning to what we already know.

Russian theorist Lev Vygotsky (1978) posited the zone of proximal
development in 1962 to address the zone (time and space) in which
learners show a readiness to learn. The zone is the level at which one

is challenged comfortably within one's ability so that the level of task difficulty is neither too difficult nor too easy (Given, 2002, p. 145). How we craft our lessons, our educational messages, and our human interactions determines if an individual is ready to learn what we have planned. We may target a group of people to learn something, but often we must tailor the lesson or message to each individual when we educate for health. The current trend is to give all learners access to the information by differentiating the lesson in more than one way, or if the lesson is designed in one way, to give learners choice in how they wish to access the information and make personal meaning and connections to the information.

Although we might really want the participants or learners to "get it" and come to understand what we know, it is not (theoretically) up to us. We must meet them halfway and be ready to honor the gap between us without crowding in or standing too far back. An exchange of information must be shared so that the learners are willing to actively pursue the information offered. This reality is perhaps one of the true challenges of the teaching–learning process. The zone of proximal development addresses the notion that certain individuals will be ready to act, others can be cued to act (and perhaps prepared for a next time), and other individuals may choose not to act this time or ever.

## Communication as a Sensory-Motor, Cognitive-Behavioral Approach

Our five senses play an impressive role in our interactions with the environment and with individuals in the environment. Interacting with the environment involves our human senses as receptors of sounds, scents, colors, light, touches, positions, and many other variables. The body organs of ears, eyes, nostrils, tongue, hands, feet, and skin act as receptors to collect the light, sound, and chemical and mechanical stimuli. Then different nerves transport the waves of sensory information into auditory, visual, olfactory, gustatory, or kinesthetic messages that the brain lobes and cortexes can interpret. The human sense organs and the different parts of the brain work together to translate incoming sensory information into integrative patterns of communication.

Although we usually form interpretations based on what our senses tell us about an object, sometimes it is useful to define a person, place, or thing by what it is *not*. For example, what if you thought about hearing as something that is unheard? Or what if you thought about seeing as something that is unseen? Or what if you thought about touching as something that is untouched? These playful exercises in language are how adults can analyze the effects of communication on human interactions. On the one hand, children and youth who are concrete thinkers will need to see it, touch it, taste it, smell it, or hear it in order to believe it. On the other hand, adults are able to think through an entire scenario for both the obvious and the hidden. When we reflect on a situation, older adolescents and adults are actually reenacting a previous situation and analyzing the outcome from more than one perspective, usually in a way that differs from what actually happened.

An area of major conflict in personal relationships is the role of speech, in which the tongue and the brain process what we say, when we say it, how we say it, and where we say it. Think about situations in which a word or phrase or sentence could have been left unsaid. Too often we express outwardly in harmful ways when we are trying to cope with a difficult situation, person, or thing.

Children who have limited language ability may communicate more freely with body gestures, actions, or mannerisms. Like words, body language can be positive or negative. Certain cultures may look, talk, or act a certain way when interacting with others; such cultural expressions of words or actions can easily be misinterpreted as rude or disrespectful by people from a different culture. Having said that, we must be mindful of the expectations we place on children and youth in certain contexts. A contextual setting of a school may need to set standards in communication for all people (i.e., the public), knowing that such restrictions or guidelines may disallow certain patterns of communication. Before these standards of behavior are communicated, professionals who work at the institution should examine a broad-based cross section of the total public represented in and by that institution. Failure to do so may result in disenfranchising or oppressing some groups by asking them to be like the dominant cultural group.

Interpersonal communication takes a great deal of practice so that the perspectives of gender, culture, and developmental readiness (i.e., age) are interwoven in our responsiveness to people. We can all think of situations when certain words or bodily expressions are intended one way but may be misinterpreted by individuals who hear them differently, see them differently, or experience them differently. As professionals, we must remember that discrepancies in communication are personal interpretations of meaning. We often cannot teach these nuances until much later in adolescence. These nuances are subtle and somewhat hidden because youngsters, and even some grown-ups, do not have the broad repertoire and skill set in communication.

Much of communication depends on our ability to access and attend to multiple sensory cues, use our thinking brains to interpret the situation, and then make a motor response through speech or actions. This is where our conscious work and explicit teaching of communication are essential with young people. For example, we should ask children and youth to follow certain steps for listening and to practice these steps daily. This means that professionals (and parents, of course) must cue kids into action. A listening action involves stopping what you are doing, looking at the person who is speaking, and hearing what the person is saying before replying with words or actions. An interactive response involves paraphrasing what was said or heard. In this simple listening process, three different responses are needed. First, on the sensory level, the eyes must see. Second, on the cognitive level, the brain must interpret the light, color, and human actions of the scene accurately and fully. Third, the person must consciously attend to the other person's comment and attempt to meet her halfway or in an interactive way so there is a win–win in the communication.

Although the individual steps of communication are somewhat easy, the overall process is complex. It's a wonder that we have any quality interactions in human communication. Many times, the communication cycle seems impossible if one person of the two is stressed, needy, or self-conscious.

The main point to take away from this discussion of communication is that both obvious and unobvious processes occur when we interact with the environment or with an individual in an environment. Our ability to integrate these processes is learned (and practiced) for a lifetime. Our human senses are the first point of contact with another person, place, or thing. When we are dealing with human interactions, we act responsibly when we give our best self to the situation. We are respectful when we honor the words and actions of the other person in a way that we would want him to honor us. So our sensory experiences evolve into our human responses of respect and responsibility. What begins as hidden patterns of sound, light, rhythm, and scents becomes a mindful response of choices to attend to certain forms of information and to ignore other forms of information. Developmentally, we then learn to interpret sensory information as a thought process that results in health-enhancing (or harmful) actions. These become more conscious decisions as children enter middle school, but they are rarely refined until adulthood.

## CHAPTER FEATURES

### Principles of Practice

• Constructivist theory encourages learners to use their background knowledge in an on-going construction of meaning, guided by their teachers who use collaborative, inquiry-based pedagogy. Constructivist approaches also seek to uncover any misconceptions or misunderstandings about health that cause inadequate or faulty thinking.

• Designs for teaching and learning require a conscious awareness of three design elements: structure, function, and aesthetics.

• All of our knowledge and thinking about health may not be functional, so we need to consciously practice (i.e., review, refine, and rethink) cognitive and behavioral responses that lead to a higher quality of life and well-being. Supportive conversations with highly competent professionals serving as healthy role models help us form our changing identities through developmental life stages.

• When educating for health, highly competent professionals will help establish conditions for learning: developmentally appropriate practices that are culturally sensitive, body–brain compatible, and health enhancing. These four conditions help us design and construct a supportive environment through which professionals in a variety of institutions and communities can educate for health.

## Teacher Voices

What follows is a teacher–coach's reflection on planning for daily instruction and thinking about the effects on 10- and 11-year-old children.

When I work at summer camps, it is helpful to do my preplanning on both a daily and weekly basis, as children come for one week and longer stints to learn gymnastics. I mentally rehearse what I am going to teach, when I am going to teach it, where in the camp I am going to teach it, why I am going to teach it, and with whom I am going to teach it EACH day. I also revisit my plan at the end of each day to make adjustments and write down notes about what actually happened.

In this reflection on planning, I will write about the many forms of planning. On the macro level of planning, there is first the preplan, followed by the actual plan of what happened.

Here's an example of how preplanning evolves. At the beginning of class each week, I look at my clipboard and chart that shows the names of my eight students for the 45-minute class and what they want to learn by the end of five classes in that week. If I look at all eight individual needs in a global sense, I see that there are patterns to my students' requests. I also observe that their plan may be beyond the scope of a week's training and that I may need to suggest a lead-up step or a different progression. For example, one gymnast wanted to learn an advanced skill but did not have the requisite lead-up skill to be able to be successful in it. In a quick exchange at the start of each class, I make sure that the student and I are in agreement with what her personal goal is for the day and what my overall plan is for her and the overall group for that day.

Effective interaction and communication with students becomes the vital link to establishing a learning environment for helping people learn. As I become a facilitator in helping each student meet her goal for the week, I do not assume that I am the only one who can teach the student. I remind my class that some of their classmates will be learning a goal similar to them, so they should watch and learn from one another. At camp, students will also spend some of their free time getting extra practice in the evening with different coaches—similar to getting help from parents on academic homework after school.

As the teacher, I am not responsible for whether a student learns her goal. Her skill development is her responsibility. However, I am able to support each student so that she can meet her goal or make adjustments to her goal. A teacher is responsible for setting different structures into a plan of action so that each student's skill is introduced and practiced throughout that week. I cannot possibly be expected to work on each person's goal each day, but my overall plan should have drills and activities that are supportive of the eight personal goals before me. In the academic classroom, this translates into cooperative structures that include solo work, small group work, and whole group activities.

It is very difficult to explain to novice teachers how one goes about learning this give and take of planning a lesson. Yet, the way to best describe the process is to balance the point of view between the curriculum and the learner and then keep the structure of time in perspective between now (the present moment) on one side and the past and future on the other side. Let's now talk about the curriculum and the learner.

When I am alone planning what I want to teach or revisiting what I actually taught at the end of the last session, I am usually writing down the "what, when, where, why, and with whom" elements of my curriculum plan. My notes usually say what content was covered, when (in what sequence), and where (in what location). I usually don't write down the why of the past but I write down the projected needs of the next session, e.g., a curriculum progression to try, a certain skill that will help this particular group of students, a particular piece of equipment or prop, and the timing of what the next session might look like. It is also important to make notes about what tasks I will need to do outside of class or equipment I will need before I see my students again.

In all my years of teaching, I rarely make notes about a particular student in my plans, because I often need the face-to-face interactions to trigger my response to that person and how to go about assisting them in the moment. The difference between planning and teaching is how I focus my energy on the story elements of "what, where, when, why, and with whom." When I am in community with my learners and am actually in the teaching act, I am usually implementing the learning process of "what, when, where, why, and with whom" from the learner's point of view. My teaching focus becomes a human act of interaction. Even though I have the content of my curriculum plan on my lesson plan and in my head, I will be people-focused when asking each student to perform a skill (what), in a certain way (why), in a certain place (where), in a group or as a solo demonstrator (with whom), and at a certain time in the class (when). These elements of the teaching story are times of engagement and occur in the present. These elements contrast to the planning tasks of teaching, which rely on the past and the future projections of the lessons.

What is the difference between objective and subjective acts of teaching? When planning, I have my lesson objectives (goals) written in my curriculum plans. While planning, I will also imagine my curriculum subject and human subjects (students) in my mind's eye. After all, if I am to educate human beings about health, I will need to understand that my subject matter is both the people and the content. However, while teaching from my lesson plan, my focus shifts to being in relationship with people in the present, so I can give them access to the content. The content can come and go from center stage throughout my lesson, but my primary responsibility is to be asking metacognitive questions like, "Is this moment working for the learner?" or "What do I need to say or do to help the learner access the information differently?" or "When, why, and with whom shall I communicate the information?" and "In which forms shall I communicate the information?"

It may be important to state the obvious here: As a teacher, I will continually set up organizational structures of lesson content, pedagogy, and people in order for my students to learn, but I will be responding and adapting to my learners as they do the learning. My ability to respond to the needs and interests of my learners depends on the articulation of individual and group goals (objective), which forms a dynamic plan of changing actions within a micro (daily) and macro (weekly) schedule. To summarize, I guide the process of learning over time by planning and structuring the learning outcomes on a daily and weekly basis (most of which is done out of contact with students) and by teaching and responding to human beings with their individual needs and interests for the session.

*Valerie Ubbes, veteran teacher–coach*

## Seeds of Growth:
## Signs, Symbols, and Patterns of Living and Learning

1. Read the following scenario and think about the role of human senses in educating for health:

> A child can determine if she needs a jacket on the playground by going outside and responding to the weather conditions by feeling the temperature on the skin and body limbs (kinesthetic cues). The child can also listen to the radio or loudspeaker for the temperature (auditory cue from sound waves), watch television for the weather report (visual and auditory cues), or simply look outside (visual cue). By reading the temperature on a thermometer (visual cue), the child uses a number (numerical cue) to determine her action. The sequential process that the student uses to make a decision to wear a jacket is first a sensory-motor and then a cognitive-behavioral response for health.

In your learning journal, write a different scenario for each habit of health—for example, nutrition, physical activity, sleep or quiet time, relationships, and hygiene. Discuss your favorite scenario with colleagues in a cooperative learning group.

2. In your learning journal, write a poem or essay that captures the essence of Nepo's quote:

> Consider the words science and conscience. Science comes from the Latin *scientia*, "to know," while conscience comes from the Latin *consciens*, "to know well." We could characterize the ability to know as retaining information and the ability to know things well as internalizing what matters. The impact of technology has extended dramatically what it is we know at a much faster rate than our ability to know things well. For to know things well requires time. But the advent of phone wires and the microchip have thrust us into a life of incredible speed, where we retain much more than we can internalize. (Nepo, 2005, p. 84)

## Web Links for Living and Learning

Take the VARK sensory learning styles inventory online at www.vark-learn. com/english/index.asp. VARK stands for visual, auditory, read/write, and kinesthetic learning styles that are sensory based. As you complete the online survey, think like a learner rather than a teacher or health professional. When you take a learning styles assessment, you need to think like a learner!

## Books for Living and Learning

In her picture book *Hands*, author and illustrator Lois Ehlert (1997) honors the many things that are made with our hands. She begins with "My father always works with his hands. He builds things in his workshop" and also talks about her mother. Make a list of all the things you do with your hands. Have a contest to see who can make the longest list in the shortest amount of time. For more ideas on what your hands can do, read the picture book *26 Big Things Small Hands Do* (Paratore, 2004) or the informational book *Made by Hand* (Goldish, 2003). You might also enjoy the picture books *Hands Are Not for Hitting* (Agassi, 2002) and *Words Are Not for Hurting* (Agassi, 2004).

Here are some of the cognitive-behavioral ways we use our hands for health and life:

Saying hello and waving good-bye

Drawing

Playing

Building

Eating and drinking

Dressing and undressing

Keeping safe

Taking care

Helping and hugging

# 4

# Ways to Know: Multiple Language Forms of Communication

Thinking, predicting, and doing are all parts of the same unfolding of sequences moving down the cortical hierarchy. "Doing" by thinking, the parallel unfolding of perception and motor behavior, is the essence of what is called goal-oriented behavior. . . . We can turn off our motor behavior, of course. I can think of seeing something without actually seeing it and I can think of going to my kitchen without actually doing so. But thinking of doing something is literally the start of how we do it.

Jeff Hawkins, *On Intelligence*

Too often, health educators advance programs and curricula—the objects of our work—instead of the people or subjects of our work. This chapter focuses on the role of identity formation while helping all human beings negotiate the multiple forms of information that promote health, wellness, and quality of life. The ability to uncover the basic signs, symbols, and patterns of information in order to form communication between human beings is the basis for language. The language of learning can be accessed by individuals and communities in search of the curriculum of life.

## Different Signs and Symbols for Language

To give people access to different ways of knowing and different forms of information, we must study the theory of multiple intelligences. Armstrong (2003) questions:

> What if Gardner had originally decided to present his ideas about multiple intelligences in the form of a song? Would anybody have listened? What if he had choreographed the concept and presented it as a dance at a large theatre hall? Would anybody have showed up? What would have happened if Gardner had originally introduced multiple intelligence theory as a series of equations or algorithms? Would anybody have cared? Would anybody have been able to figure them out? (p. 3)

According to Armstrong (2003), Gardner drew from several different disciplines to determine his theory of multiple intelligences, such as anthropology, developmental psychology, animal physiology, brain research, cognitive science, and biographies of exceptional individuals. "Taken in this manner, MI theory serves as an important impetus toward fundamental reforms of our educational system, leading to a re-evaluation of those subjects typically taught in school, with increased emphasis placed on the arts, nature, physical culture, and other topics traditionally limited to the periphery of the curriculum" (p. 4).

What happens when we use multiple intelligences as an organizer or mental framework for learning? The learning power of multiple intelligences is that you and your learners can use and integrate a variety of symbol systems into a richer, more authentic study. As you educate for health, the more you can integrate a variety of symbol systems (e.g., words, pictures, numbers, body language, rhythms, and environmental cues), the deeper and more well-rounded your students will become in their understanding and meaning making. Specifically, your investigations of health-related topics, concepts, and skills form language patterns that are building blocks to more sophisticated forms of communication. You can increase learning outcomes by exploring health information through different language elements and disseminating it through different communication formats (e.g., print, nonprint, and broadcast resources). When young people actively design or implement these different language elements through active engagement—instead of passively receiving health messages—there is greater potential for learning.

According to Ubbes and Ward (2007), health educators serve as gatekeepers for students as they access information, products, and services. A novice professional becomes an expert professional when he has the competence to represent health-related information in multiple language elements and communication formats. Table 4.1 shows different communication media aligned with four of the eight multiple intelligences. Sample media formats are also provided. In the information age, we need to know how to educate for health using a variety of communication media in different formats. So much of our positive and negative messages come to young people through these formats. However, as you will learn in chapter 7, developing a relational pedagogy is a very important

## Table 4.1 Communication Media and Formats

| Multiple intelligence | Communication media | Media formats |
| --- | --- | --- |
| Verbal linguistic | Spoken | Storytelling, speeches, conversations in one or more languages |
| | Broadcast | Newscast, talk radio, talk show in one or more languages |
| | Print | Newspapers, leaflets, flyers, pamphlets, brochures, books |
| | Recorded | Books on tape, monologues |
| Visual spatial | Artifact | Museum exhibit, juried show |
| | Recorded | Photograph, video, digital video disk |
| Musical rhythmical and bodily kinesthetic | Performance | Concert, rehearsal, practice |
| | Recorded | Compact disk, audiocassette, MP3, radio, television |

goal in health education, because we are educating human beings for an enhanced quality of life. Technology can and does enhance our lives, but too many young people and professionals live in a virtual world instead of having the real "lived" experience of well-being.

As human beings, we use words and body language when communicating or expressing ourselves. In communication theory, we tend to use the words *verbal* and *nonverbal* as a way to categorize our language patterns. Unfortunately, when we choose to label our words as verbal and all other patterns as nonverbal, we isolate the ways many people access and share information in the world. Although our thoughts and our ability to speak make us humans when compared with other life forms of plants and animals, we must also realize the limits of such distinctions. For example, humans who are mute cannot speak, humans who are blind cannot see, and humans who are limited in physical abilities cannot move in traditional ways. The special ways these people communicate, although limited in one or more human senses, are vital to how they make sense of the world. As teachers, we must be mindful of the different forms of communication (e.g., spoken and written language, sign language, and Braille, to name a few).

## Structure, Function, and Aesthetic Forms of Language

We must be especially sensitive about the combination of communication forms that individuals use to access and share information. Typically, our words and actions communicate what we are thinking and feeling inside. Our choice of words is important—especially words that shape and fashion the world to make it a better place. And depending on how words are structured and formed, they can be either encouraging or discouraging. From a design perspective, not all words are functional. It takes courage for humans to find their voices in the world and learn how to contribute their points of view, so teachers serve as bridges to those communication forms, whether they are shared in words or in actions of different symbol systems. Table 4.2 organizes the elements of language as signs, symbols, and semiotic patterns. Another word for semiotics is *semantics*. The word *semantics* can be defined as the study of meaning in language. Semiotic patterns for the basic elements of language include words, pictures, numbers, body language, rhythms, and environmental cues. These language elements form different communication types or genre.

It is vitally important to give people access to a variety of ways to communicate. Words are important in the world, even prized over other expressions in certain professions. However, one's progression in

Table 4.2    **Elements of Language: Signs, Symbols, and Semiotic Patterns**

| Multiple intelligence | Signs and symbols | Patterns | Elements of language | Communication types or genre |
|---|---|---|---|---|
| Verbal linguistic | Punctuation, letters of the alphabet | Words, phrases, sentences, paragraphs, stories | Spoken words | Conversation, debate, discussion, dialogue |
| | | | Written words | Short story, novel, biography, prose, autobiography, poetry, lyrics, quotes, narrative, expository text |
| Visual spatial | Colors, icons, space | Graphics, light, pictures | Pictures | Drawing, sketching, painting, etching, printmaking, sculpture, calligraphy, computer graphics |
| Logical mathematical | Lines, shapes, vectors, angles, numerals, logical operators, mathematical notation | Calculations, algorithms, logical arguments, proofs | Numbers | Algebra, geometry, calculus, statistics, trigonometry, functions |
| Bodily kinesthetic | Nonverbal expressions, body positions, kinesthetic pressure | Body posture, body mechanics, human senses, movement | Body language | Sport, dance, theater (mime), exercise |
| Musical rhythmical | Musical notation, key signature, time signature, stanza | Measure, movement phrase, song, melody, sounds, rhythmical beats | Rhythms | Rap, classical, country, baroque, hip hop, rock, rhythm and blues, pop, jazz |
| Naturalist environmental | Flora, fauna, weather, elements (rocks, minerals, water, fire) | Nature, biomes | Environmental cues | Biology, zoology, botany, chemistry, physics, astronomy, geology |

accessing and using dance, art, music, sport, exercise, theater, or other communication types or genre increases the opportunity for designs that educate for health.

Why do designs that educate for health need to employ words and other forms of communication? In terms of development, young people first learn to crawl, walk, and talk, although the walking and talking patterns vary from individual to individual. At certain points of development, the coordination and integration of words with body expressions move from being cute at age 2 to practical at age 12. Sometimes the words tell the story, and other times the actions tell the real story. As we support young people in their development, we enable them to find many ways to communicate what they know and will come to know in their next stage of development.

Indeed, although the media continue to manipulate the structure, function, and aesthetics of communication, young people are not as coordinated in their response in terms of what to say, how to say it, or what actions are appropriate for what words. It takes time and a great deal of guidance from parents, caregivers, and teachers to help children and youth communicate effectively.

When we educate for health, we must learn to compose our messages in a combination of words, pictures, numbers, body language, rhythms, and environmental cues. Introducing young people to these multiple signs and symbol systems enables them to gain access to "who" they are and "what" language forms are meaningful to them. We can encourage people with health-promoting messages so they are cued for positive action. If they choose not to hear or heed messages in words, then we need to employ other language forms—from both natural and virtual environments—to inspire them. In short, the theory of multiple intelligences promotes multiple representations so that humans have greater access to their life potential.

## Intelligence Defined

Intelligence represents a person's biological and psychological potential. Gardner (1985) defines intelligence as "the ability to solve problems, or create products, which are valued in one or more cultural settings" (p. x). Gardner interpreted his understanding of intelligences differently from Alfred Binet and Theodore Simon, who created one of the first ways to measure intelligence in schools. In 1905, the French government asked Binet and Simon to distinguish slow learners from the general population. After being revised and standardized at Stanford University in 1916, the Stanford-Binet Intelligence Scale became a source for assessing an individual's intelligence by an intelligence quotient (IQ), which has been used to predict school success (Malow-Iroff, Benhar, & Martin, 2005).

Blythe and Gardner (1990) claim that "MI theory challenges the viability of standardized, machine-scored, multiple-choice assessments, which by their very nature appraise students' knowledge through the filter of the linguistic and logical-mathematical intelligences" (p. 33). Instead, humans use a profile of multiple intelligences to represent what they know, from words to pictures to bodily expressions, to name a few.

A principle of multiple intelligences theory is that humans often show a preference for or ability in a few or more intelligences, but each individual has a personal profile of eight intelligences to varying degrees. According to Blythe and Gardner, "Every normal individual possesses varying degrees of each of these intelligences, but the ways in which intelligences combine and blend are as varied as the faces and the personalities of individuals. . . . MI theory emphasizes the highly individualized ways in which people learn" (p. 36).

We can refine our intelligences through experience and practice. An inquiry process allows us to fashion products and performances of understanding that are unique to our multiple intelligences profile. The multiple intelligences are named and defined as follows:

- Verbal linguistic (V/L) intelligence is the ability to recognize, use, and understand the signs, symbols, and patterns of words.

- Visual spatial (V/S) intelligence is the ability to recognize, use, and understand the signs, symbols, and patterns of pictures.

- Logical mathematical (L/M) intelligence is the ability to recognize, use, and understand the signs, symbols, and patterns of numbers and reasoning.

- Bodily kinesthetic (B/K) intelligence is the ability to recognize, use, and understand the patterns of body language and movement forms.

- Musical rhythmical (M/R) intelligence is the ability to recognize, use, and understand the signs, symbols, and patterns of rhythm and music.

- Naturalist environmental (N/E) intelligence is the ability to recognize, use, and understand the signs, symbols, and patterns of nature and the environment.

Two other intelligences are named as people intelligences:

- Intrapersonal introspective intelligence is the ability to know and understand oneself.

- Interpersonal social intelligence is the ability to know and understand other people.

Gardner (1995) states that "students secure a sense of what it is like to be an expert when they behold that a teacher can represent knowledge in a number of different ways and discover that they themselves are also capable of more than a single representation of a specified content." I believe the real benefit of using multiple intelligences in teaching and learning seems to be the ways people can gain access to different language elements.

# Domain-Specific Information and Expert Performance

Achievement in all domains is acquired during an extended period of training and development (Ericsson, 2005). To be good at something, deliberate practice is necessary at all levels of performance (e.g., novice, intermediate, expert).

Human information processing theory (Newell & Simon, 1972) assumes that exceptional performance results when knowledge and skills are acquired through experience. This theory suggests that expertise is basically our ability to access a greater vocabulary of patterns and chunks of information in a domain. With experience, more complex and sophisticated patterns gradually accumulate.

Ericsson (2005) suggests that skilled learning is more than accumulating knowledge. Deliberate practice activities must be tightly coordinated and focus sequentially on improving one specific aspect of performance at a time. There is a complex mechanism for mediating learning. Feedback is needed with deliberate practice.

# Role of Human Senses in Information Processing

We use our five senses to respond to different forms of information. Our sensory organs (ears, eyes, skin, tongue, and nose) receive messages from human interactions, from media sources, and from nature. This sensory information is then carried by different pathways into the brain for processing. The brain interprets communication signs and symbols as patterns of sound, sight, touch, taste, and smell, but we must attend to these in a conscious way in order to make sense of them. To be sure, unlimited sensory information is available to our sensory organs. Fortunately, our human senses use selective attention (e.g., selective listening, selective seeing) to process the signs, symbols, and patterns that can be used to communicate what we know. In teaching, we are able to choose which senses our learners use to help them attend to the lesson. When this is explicit, we say that we got our learners' attention.

Although it may not be taught as a complex pattern of sight, sound, and touch, listening includes many human senses. Young children must be taught how to listen effectively. An effective listener stops what he or she is doing, looks at the speaker with focused attention, and listens for the information being presented before responding with words and body mannerisms or actions. In this example, the eyes, body, ears, and tongue are busy receiving and processing information from one person to another. When no response is given after a speaker has finished, there is an incredible loss of understanding in this one-way exchange. When humans have a variety of ways in which to respond and fail to do so, it is interpreted as limited communication skills. Children and grown-ups have the "response-ability" to acknowledge one another when spoken to in words, touched by body language, or greeted through nonverbal gestures. Failure to do so creates an information gap.

## Role of Language and Literacy in Educating for Health

As one who will educate for health, you need to make meaning through the multiple signs, symbols, and patterns of language. Language is made up of multiple forms of information, each represented by different signs, symbols, and patterns for communicating. Since communication is a basic concept and skill in education, we can explore the relationships between the concepts of communication, education, and health as a way to seek quality of life. In this context, language can be defined beyond the spoken word, although written and printed words are often the sole basis for literacy.

The theory of multiple intelligences identifies the signs, symbols, and patterns of eight different intelligences. I refer to these signs, symbols, and patterns as the common elements of language that we use to communicate what we know in the world. We communicate in the language of words, pictures, numbers, body language, rhythms, and environmental cues. We can reduce each of these languages to a simpler form that may be more developmentally appropriate. The verbal linguistic intelligence can be reduced to having word sense, being word smart, and then having linguistic intelligence. If a child has word sense, she can listen to and recite the alphabet and say the letters aloud, make simple word utterances at first, then form sentences using verbal (linguistic) speech. During the later preschool years, she is able to recognize the different letters of the alphabet and read basic words by repetition. She can also write the letters of her name and even copy certain words that are placed in front of her. Eventually, having a "sense" of words (i.e., word sense) evolves into being word smart. The child can now decode the words on a page or billboard and recognize certain words or phrases, eventually completing sentences to make up paragraphs. The letters of spoken and written words are symbols that make up a language; the punctuation marks on a page are the signs that are read to form linguistic patterns, either read silently or read aloud.

When we educate for health, we use many spoken (verbal) and written messages to communicate health information. These messages can be either read by children or heard by children. This requires information processing that begins with the human senses receiving and translating neurochemical signals, which then are interpreted by the brain. The goal of semiotics in educating for health is to realize the myriad ways a child is able to make sense of words (e.g., word sense), then to show how to use words in appropriate and effective ways (e.g., word smart). Eventually, when these developmental stages are refined through adequate trial and error using spoken and written word forms, we can acknowledge the child's verbal linguistic intelligences.

Expertise in language could mean that a child learns to speak different cultural languages, including different ways to write the signs and symbols of that language. In cultural contexts, a child could learn English and Spanish and a host of other human languages. If I were to walk you through a similar exercise using the bodily kinesthetic intelligence, I would mention the value of sign language by first teaching the manual alphabet as communicated by hand signals. See if you can do this developmentally appropriate staging of bodily kinesthetic intelligence. Can you give examples of how a child has a sense of his body? What would represent his ability to demonstrate body sense? How is the child able to be body smart? What are some examples of this? And finally, as the child grows in sophistication and refinement through trial and error, what repertoire would he model for bodily kinesthetic intelligence?

Bodily kinesthetic intelligence is especially important because our human senses are key pathways for sensing our bodies and the world around us. And the human senses are the ways we access all information to be perceived and learned. Thus, our bodily kinesthetic intelligence determines how we learn through information processing (as initiated and accessed through our human senses). Our bodily kinesthetic intelligence plays a key role in how we educate for health so that we learn to share health-related information through multiple modalities and sensory-motor pathways. This means that as we educate for health, we must know how to present information with a variety of signs, symbols, and patterns through different genres and multiple formats and channels.

## Literacy and Health

Literacy is the highest form of human accomplishment. The ability to read and write makes us uniquely human and separates us from other life forms, including from each other, depending on one's level of education. As we educate for health, we must be mindful of the health disparities among those who can access, read, and comprehend the printed word.

The World Health Organization recently named health literacy as a global priority (Wilson, 2003). Literacy predicts an individual's health status more strongly than age, income, employment status, education level, and racial or ethnic group (Partnership for Clear Health Communication, 2003). Therefore, we are wise to educate for health with an emphasis on health literacy.

Health literacy is the "capacity of an individual to obtain, interpret, and understand basic health information and services and the competence to use such information and services in ways which are health-enhancing" (Joint Committee on National Health Education Standards, 2007). Health literacy can be advanced through education and health strategies across the life span. However, there are critical foundation years for promoting health and disease prevention during early and middle childhood.

As you read this text, I am hopeful that you will learn the language of education and health at the same time, especially any language that defines the discipline of health education. Until you can unpack the language for this trip and begin to use it in your daily studies, you will only passively participate as a spectator on the journey. By joining a community of learners along the way, and having access to the terminology for thinking, writing, and speaking about your experiences, you will be more likely to refine your professional goals now, rather than waiting until you get your first professional position. Just as your human identity is defined by multiple dimensions of health, there are multiple forms of communication (albeit intelligences) that will enable you to educate for health. Knowing one way to communicate makes you a novice. But knowing multiple ways to communicate makes you an expert who can give others access to important health-related messages for life and learning.

Prior and Gerard (2004) also suggest the following:

> Environmental print is one of the first sources of reading material for young children and serves as soil for the roots of literacy. . . . Environmental print helps children to understand how written language is organized and used. Early notions about print, directionality, function, and letter sounds take shape as children realize that the print in their everyday world holds meaning and serves important purposes. (p. iv)

Enz (2003) defines environmental print as "print that occurs in real-life contexts—the signs, billboards, logos, and functional print that saturate a child's world" (cited from Prior & Gerard, 2004, p. iv). It can also occur as product labels, print on cereal boxes and food packages, and store signs. Prior and Gerard (2004) further describe environmental print:

The capital letter *K* in the Kmart department store sign and in the Circle K grocery store sign are similar—red uppercase letters—yet children know the two separate logos because of the surrounding graphic and context clues that come before and after the big red K. Young children search context in order to read the Kmart logo. The blue background of the Kmart logo is quite different from the red circle background of the Circle K logo. Syntactic clues are internalized as grammar rules and word order emerges from reading environmental print. The fast-food restaurant name Burger King cannot be read as King Burger correctly. All the linguistic cueing systems—graphophonics, semantics, and syntax—work together powerfully in the young child's reading of environmental print (p. 4).

Simmons, Gunn, Smith, and Kameenui (1994) have found that phonemic awareness—the awareness of the size of sound units in phonemes, syllables, and words—is the most recognizable characteristic of proficient readers. Prior and Gerard (2004) remind us that "while the identification of letters and sounds is essential for reading success, reading is, first and foremost, a meaning-making process. The ultimate goal is the comprehension of text" (p. 2). Further, "Speaking, listening, reading, and writing are not separate skills acquired independently of each other. Children learn all meaningful communication by using it purposefully in social contexts" (p. 5).

## Health Communication

Understanding information requires human reasoning known as information processing, which is mediated by the body and brain. Information enters the brain as sensory data in the form of light or sound waves and in the form of kinesthetic pressure, temperature, and positional sensations through mechanoreceptors in the skin and body joints. These sensory data are recognized (perceived) by the brain as sensory-motor responses that can then inform our cognitive-behavioral actions.

Across all languages, humans use the following elements to communicate: words as written text and spoken language; images, pictures, icons, and graphics; numbers and sequences; nonverbal body language, facial expressions, and movement; rhythm and music; and environmental cues from the natural world.

We use each element to communicate and construct meaning through a language. These subtextual elements either remain as implicit subjective thoughts or become explicit communication that is shared in different ways. When we interpret these language elements into a pattern, communication results.

Communication, which is related to community through the root word *common*, involves the transmittal of information through various channels. Elements of language (e.g., signs, symbols, and patterns) serve as a metalanguage for helping us communicate with one another. According to the theory of multiple intelligences (Gardner, 1983; Lazear, 1999; Berk, 2001; Ubbes, 2004), humans are both self-smart (e.g., intrapersonal introspective, leading to self-identity) and people smart (e.g., interpersonal social, which includes a social construction of meaning in a dynamic environment) (Vygotsky, 1962, 1978). There is continual interaction between the human self in private and personal spheres, including self as a member of a public community and society.

# A Developmental Perspective of Language as Play

Play is categorized as a spontaneous, sensory process that is intrinsic for young children. It is rewarding all by itself and has no ultimate goals. Play is a life space and experience where children learn culture, rules, conflict resolution, and how to reconstruct play. Television results in inactive play instead of interaction. There is a balance needed between structured play and spontaneous play.

Erikson (1950) identified three levels of play in childhood: autocosmic play as a self-world of waving hands and feet; microcosmic play as a small world of dolls, stuffed animals, and other toys as a surrogate for human companionship; and macrocosmic play as a large-world mastery of tools (e.g., pencils and crayons, scissors, computer).

According to Prior and Gerard (2004, p. 14), play is very important for early language development. "Play with language and language in play" is especially important. Play with language begins for the infant as sound play and manipulation of vocalization (e.g., phonological elements of language). After an infant understands the "sound system of language," young children develop two-word utterances. Language in play uses pretend play, which "helps children to plan play episodes, negotiate and carry out play roles, and talk about play events." During this time, children transform their identities and the identities of others (Fein, 1981).

Prior and Gerard (2004) contend that Vygotsky's zone of proximal development theory, which is discussed in chapter 3, helped liberate children from real or actual constraints in play:

> Fantasy allows young children to separate objects and their meaning or to substitute one object for another object. . . . Representational play . . . prepare[s] children for later abstract thinking and use of literacy symbols. Blocks become a skyscraper, a desk becomes a

racecar, and a ruler becomes a magic wand. The young child's representational thought processes in play allow a picture in a book to represent reality and then allow written words to represent the pictures. Make-believe and the fantasy of play are intimately linked to reading and writing in the later years. (p. 13)

Language helps children to organize their thinking. . . . Language bridges the gap between action and thinking; it is one of the most significant areas of development during the preschool, kindergarten, and primary years. Similarly, motor skills, social roles, vocabulary, story sequence, and peer relationships develop in play for young children. Play is the integrated space for learning across these domains. (pp. 12-13)

## Conceptual Design

The Committee on Learning Research and Educational Practice (National Research Council, 2002) has acknowledged that experts draw on a rich information base in order to transform facts into usable knowledge. To develop competence in an area of learning, learners must merge a deep factual knowledge with a strong conceptual framework. The National Research Council (2002) states: "A conceptual framework allows experts to organize information into meaningful patterns and store it hierarchically in memory to facilitate retrieval for problem solving" (p. 2).

In her book *Concept-Based Curriculum and Instruction: Teaching Beyond the Facts*, Lynn Erickson (1998) states that concepts meet the following criteria: a one- or two-word mental construct that is broad, abstract, timeless, and universal. A concept bridges disciplines, and a conceptual lens forces thinking to the integration level. Students see patterns and connections at the conceptual level if we let them define what they see in their own words, with their own examples. Without a conceptual lens, a topic of study remains at a lower cognitive level, and students seek to memorize the facts related to the topic. Table 4.3 shows a sample of concepts that can bridge disciplines to form transdisciplinary macroconcepts. These concepts (e.g., change, time, structure, balance, movement, boundaries, cycle, and relationship) can often be found in health education lessons and curricula.

I believe we can make a more concerted effort to use transdisciplinary concepts in middle school health education and beyond by investigating their connections to habits of health and habits of mind. Because only one-third of eighth graders are typically able to use abstract thinking (Van Hoose, Strahan, & L'Esperance, 2001), I encourage teaching these abstract concepts in concrete ways, with hands-on props and models, through repetition and bridging activities to interdisciplinary units in schools that promote inquiry-based investigations.

# Table 4.3    Sample of Transdisciplinary Concepts

| Macroconcepts | Sample connections to disciplines |
|---|---|
| Change | • Some teens change from calm to stressed when a teacher moves the class schedule ahead by five minutes.<br>• The man reached into his jeans for some pocket change.<br>• Change is often symbolized by the Greek letter delta, or a triangle. |
| Time | • The globe is divided into different time zones.<br>• When the second hand goes around the clock one time, a minute has passed.<br>• Young people need to make time for 9 1/4 hours of sleep in a 24-hour day. |
| Structure | • Skeletal bones structure the human body so organs can be protected in different cavities.<br>• The new building structure collapsed in the inclement weather.<br>• Humans often structure their schedules with too many activities. |
| Balance | • The dancer balanced on one foot in her theatrical performance.<br>• The balance tipped when the suitcases were placed on the scales to be weighed.<br>• Humans need a daily diet that balances six major nutrients. |
| Movement | • The opening movement of the sonata was played with gusto.<br>• There was a slight movement of waves as the diver dove into the water.<br>• Physical movement can help reduce our perception of stress. |
| Boundaries | • The city boundaries were being challenged by legal debate.<br>• Teens cross boundaries in order to seek new information, which may pose high health risks.<br>• The soccer ball crossed the boundaries of the sideline. |
| Cycle | • The cycle of supply and demand often determines the success of a recycling program.<br>• The child rode his bicycle with the traffic to obey transportation rules.<br>• The human body has many hormonal cycles based on light and darkness. |
| Relationship | • The relationship between ideas in the first and second sentence was not obvious.<br>• The brass and woodwinds played in a harmonic relationship with one another.<br>• Human relationships are vitally important to a sense of identity and belonging. |

# Design Problem Solving in Educating for Health

Problem solving is an ongoing thought process that professionals use to approach questions of design. When assessing the structure, function, and aesthetics (quality) of health education materials, lessons, and curricula, numerous problems surface. In health education, we want young people to come to know, understand, and value their bodies and brains. In health communication and literacy, we want teachers, parents, and caregivers to understand the body of knowledge that is available to educate for health. Children and youth can get a jump start on life if they are given access to health-related information in multiple forms and intelligences during their formative years.

In some respects, we have reduced design to a problem-solving, inquiry-based approach in education for only a few select individuals, namely the best and the brightest. But inquiry-based education can still use fresh and novel problem-naming, problem-framing, and problem-solving approaches. *Problem solving* is a term that ushered in a new era of thinking about intellectual ability, spurred on by J.P. Guilford in his 1949 address to the American Psychological Association.

In his seminal 1950 paper, Guilford made a distinction between two different cognitive processes: convergent thinking and divergent thinking. Convergent thinking focuses on recognizing the familiar and preserving what is already known. The function of convergent thought is to acquire factual knowledge and perfect what is already known. On the other hand, divergent thinking involves the production of novelty and variability, leading to multiple answers. The function of divergent thought is to develop new ways of knowing, including changing what is known through imagination and invention.

In his book *Creativity in Education and Learning: A Guide for Teachers and Educators*, Cropley (2001) insists that novelty, like memorization, can be fostered in everybody, not just the chosen few. He suggests that schools, universities, businesses, and families need to promote the creative potential of individuals. This includes finding new approaches to old problems with a fresh perspective.

Cropley (2001) defines cognitive structures as "internal representations of the external world that are built up on the basis of experience—they reflect and summarize the accumulated experiences of the individual and are stored in memory" (p. 29). These structures can be organized as patterns, categories, or networks of information that are interpreted by the body senses and brain through information processing.

As previously mentioned, in his definition of multiple intelligences, Gardner (1993) states that intelligence is the ability to solve problems or create products that are valued in one or more cultures. To solve such problems, an individual may draw on what is known and conventional or unknown and novel. According to Gardner, as long as the resulting signs, symbols, and patterns lead to outcomes that are valued by a culture or organized group of individuals, then the effect is intelligent behavior. Said another way, the results of the problem solving must be communicated and then subsequently valued. Cropley (2001) suggests that creative achievements may have both tangible and intangible elements, with some results seen in concrete objects and others in abstract symbol systems. "Every far fetched, outrageous, or preposterous idea or every astonishing act of non-conformity" is not to be deemed creative. A crucial property of creativity is that it is deemed ethical and leads to positive intentions (p. 15).

According to Gardner (1997), a person with expertise can conceptualize multiple representations of a problem:

> Frequently, breakthroughs occur because the individual has been able to conceive of familiar problems or challenges in a new way. . . . He or she can think about the problem in a number of ways, particularly ways that have not previously been brought to bear on that problem. The more that an individual can make use of his unique strengths in attacking a problem, the more likely that he will arrive at an approach that holds special . . . promise for illuminating that problem. (p. 149)

## Design for Action Potentials, Action Plans, and Action Research

As one who will educate for health, you will need to understand the word *action*. Action potentials allow your neurons to fire and encode information into memory pathways for representing information in more than one way. The more representations you have for a particular health topic, concept, or skill, the greater your schema for that information. Hence, your expertise (i.e., background knowledge) is dependent on the number of neuronal connections in your nervous system and how often you consciously revisit the information in your thoughts or actions.

Table 4.4 shows how we organize knowledge when we educate for health. Declarative knowledge is what we know; procedural knowledge is what we do; and contextual knowledge is what we know and do in a particular context or situation. Declarative, procedural, and contextual knowledge are ways to structure and organize the elements of knowledge when we make plans to educate for health. When we want young people to know more schema about their health and well-being, we organize our lessons by facts, topics, concepts, generalizations, principles, models, and theories to help them learn. When we want young people to practice more schema for health-enhancing skills and behaviors, we organize

Table 4.4  **Structure of Knowledge**

| Meaning or etymology | Elements of knowledge |
|---|---|
| Declarative knowledge: *to know* | Types of declarative knowledge:<br>• Facts, topics, concepts, generalizations, principles, models, and theories |
| Procedural knowledge: *to do* | Types of procedural knowledge:<br>• Skills, strategies, techniques, methods, procedures, and processes<br>• *Method* comes from the Greek *meta* (beyond, after) + *hodos* (way), hence after the regular way, following the prescribed or systematic way. The Greek *meta* also gives us such words as *metamorphosis, metaphor, metacognitive, meta-analysis, metabolism, metacarpals,* and *metatarsus* (the part of the foot after the tarsus, or ankle) |
| Contextual knowledge: *to know and do original work in a particular place at a certain time with certain people while using specific tools, props, or pedagogies* | Conditions of contextual knowledge:<br>• Place, location, or setting<br>• Timing<br>• People<br>• Tools, props, or pedagogies |

our lessons by skills, strategies, techniques, methods, procedures, and processes. When we want young people to practice integrating what they know with what they do for daily health and well-being, we organize our lessons with different places, timing, people, and pedagogies in mind. This helps kids develop more neuronal pathways and more efficient firing patterns through repeated exposure and practice in different contexts.

When we consciously plan to focus on contextual knowledge, we often need to interact with other professionals, parents, and community leaders so we can form a supportive network of humans who will continue to cue kids with similar words, pictures, numbers, body language, rhythms, and environmental cues that are linked to health-enhancing topics, concepts, and skills. We all need to use language forms with recognizable patterns to communicate with young people.

As you educate for health, you will especially need to understand and promote cues to action that help you and others practice the five habits of health and five habits of mind (figure 4.1) on a daily basis. It takes lots of practice (and often cues from significant people in our lives) to practice these five behaviors (i.e., habits of health) and five cognitive skills (i.e., habits of mind) each day. But if we consider our lesson plans as action plans, we can educate for health more often and help young people practice these actions for being healthy and well.

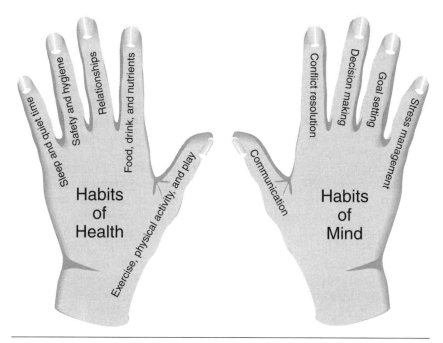

**Figure 4.1**   Habits of health and habits of mind.

When you learn in chapter 5 to write action plans for health in the form of lesson plans, you will be integrating what you know with what you do to educate for health. You can also conduct action research in your internships and student teaching to determine if your teaching has made a difference in the learning outcomes of your students. We need to move beyond the practice of only a few individuals thinking about the question of improvement. Students need to learn how to learn, learn how to plan, and learn how to research and review their own progress toward their habits of health and habits of mind.

## Habits of Health and Habits of Mind as Possibilities for Healthful Practices

I have chosen a model of habits of health and habits of mind using two hand graphics because they are related to the human body. During child and adolescent development, learners use concrete thinking to make decisions. To produce skilled movements for habits of health, there needs to be repetition of motor patterns. To produce skilled thinking for habits of mind, there needs to be repetition of cognitive patterns.

I love how the word *recognition* can be analyzed as *re + cognition*. When we are cognizant of repeating signs, symbols, and patterns of communication, such semiotics may increase our readiness to act on the health-related messages. *Read-i-ness* can also be analyzed to mean the ability to read words on a page or billboard, read a picture on a poster or health pamphlet, read numbers on a food label, read the body language of a peer, and so forth. Educating for health involves preparing people to recognize and use multiple signs, symbols, and patterns of language to increase their readiness to act on their changing understanding of health messages and resources. Ultimately, our actions need to lead to habits of health and habits of mind on a daily basis.

As indicated in the last chapter on establishing a constructivist approach to teaching and learning, teachers and students can be co-designers of the educational experience. These collaborative teaching–learning experiences can also be found in standards-based environments. The wise professional creates a space for student voice and choice in his or her own learning. Such opportunities create a unity between what the student wants to know and what the student needs to know based on the school curriculum and disciplinary standards that teachers use as guidelines for their action plans. Sometimes teachers do not think that students can be co-planners in a standards-based environment, but the following assumption tells us why this may be important: When educating for health, you will have very little control over whether a student will wash hands, effectively manage a conflict with a peer, eat fruits and vegetables at lunch, or arrive to school with adequate sleep. Therefore, the curriculum standards for health education focus on the personal and social skills that enable students to think about and practice health-related behaviors in school, home, and community contexts.

Indeed, your cues to action and environmental supports for helping children practice health-related skills and behaviors at school are very important. It is essential that you structure both planned and incidental learning episodes for health education in your classroom. You should also construct some homework assignments that bridge health education from school to home, home to community, and community to school. This three-way interactive network ensures that the grown-ups in young people's lives know what kids are learning in schools.

This is idealistic, however. Unless the health education curriculum is disseminated from one location to another, there is no way of sharing the list of skills that kids need to practice from place to place. In a best-case scenario, the skills for listening effectively, managing stress, setting goals, resolving conflict, communicating with assertion, and using refusal skills effectively should be printed in multiple places in the school–home–community network. Such health communication can be initiated by teachers who educate for health and then sustained by caring parents who work in partnership with the school and community.

With cues for action coming from the grown-ups and hopefully peers in students' lives, we can establish a supportive web of connectivity for the important PRE-vention work of kids. In this context, *PRE* serves as an acronym for predisposing factors, reinforcing factors, and enabling factors, which inform the educational and environmental phases of the PRECEDE–PROCEED model of public health planning (Green & Kreuter, 2005). These factors, described in figure 4.2, show the complexity of determining whether an individual will choose a healthy behavior, known in this text as a habit of health. In short, the predisposing factors refer to the individual's attitudes, beliefs, values, and perceptions of the health habit; the enabling factors refer to the home, school, and community resources available to the individual; and the reinforcing factors refer to the amount of encouragement (or discouragement) from significant people in the individual's life to choose a habit of health. These three factors are interrelated and are associated with practicing positive, preventive health behaviors or not (Bonaguro, 1981). Predisposing factors are needed to motivate a health behavior, and reinforcing factors determine whether a habit of health will continue to be practiced or be extinguished. For a further explanation of these factors of prevention, see Wooley (1995).

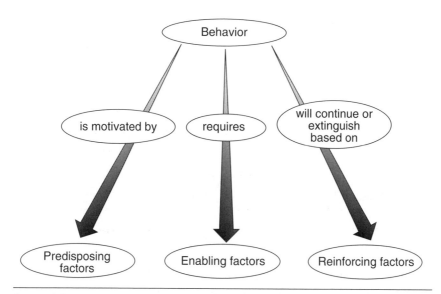

**Figure 4.2**   PRE-vention model to solve health-related behaviors.

Reprinted, by permission, from S. Wooley, 1995, "Behavior mapping: A tool for identifying priorities for health education curricula and instruction," *Journal of Health Education* 26(4): 202.

PRE-vention work is a form of problem solving. As a teacher, if you fail to cue students for hand washing before meals or after being on the playground, you are not being supportive of health education. If you drink a can of soda while you are teaching, you are not modeling health-enhancing behaviors related to nutrition or hydration. If you do not structure learning time for health education, you are not giving children and youth practice time to refine their personal skills of decision making and goal setting or their social skills of communication and conflict resolution. The modeling of voice and choice begins with your comfort level in working with the National Health Education Standards as guidelines. In a metaphorical sense, a teacher does not need to be hopeless or helpless in how to structure health-enhancing experiences for children and youth. The process of guiding and cuing young people with health-related choices within a healthy environment is very similar to how a teacher functions with a standards-based set of guidelines for health education—or any discipline for that matter.

## Problems of PreK-12 Health Curriculum

Since few if any of us receive health education courses *every* year in preK-12 schooling during our developmental years, the subtle message is that we all "know" about health and can learn it either on our own or as we go along. Over the years, without an explicit and consistent study of health in an educational context, we learn to position health as a subtext in our lives. It's there, but it's just part of life.

I have noticed that young people are often taught to overlook and *not* attend to their basic health needs because of the way schools and homes are structured around adult needs. This structuring of the school curriculum and school day unfortunately limits the number of minutes that children and youth receive focused health instruction between the ages of 5 and 18. Although some kids get supportive and nurturing messages from home, the print and broadcast media continue to project unhealthy and unbalanced messages to a younger and younger audience. These media messages in the community and on the way to and from school each day are greater in number and frequency than the health-related messages scheduled in the school curriculum. This, then, becomes a critical problem in society when conflicting messages are heard and then practiced by children who are concrete, hands-on learners.

Wellness and illness messages must be studied within many academic disciplines, not just health education, because healthful and harmful lifestyles permeate our personal lives and need to be discussed in multiple contexts. This important discussion about healthful and harmful messages should not be omitted from our professional lives either. In ongoing disciplinary discussions of educational theory and practices, health issues must be promoted by all teachers and administrators. We can no longer afford to rely on health education and physical education teachers to carry the burden of educating for health in a few random years of preK-12 schooling.

The cycle of curriculum review, often not equitable for health education, physical education, music, and art, has remained under the jurisdiction of busy administrators who can limit updates and progressive policies to "core subjects" versus "encore subjects" within the school community. For example, many administrators and policy makers who come through their own professional preparation course work and internships still do not learn about health education in a planned, sequential way. In a pressure-filled environment of high-stakes testing, decisions are made by default instead of in open discussions with teachers, who when empowered with opportunities for adult discourse, can help solve problems in critical and creative ways.

Teachers are more connected to the hearts of young people because education is central to their lives, and they can tell you candidly what works and what could work better. Administrators often share these connections of the heart, but their agendas are more program, curricula, and policy driven around the core subjects. I remind you here and frequently throughout this text that health education is one area in the school community where we focus on people as the sole motivation for learning. A curriculum of health and wellness is not about plants, animals, places, or things; it is a curriculum about people who need to practice healthful skills and behaviors across their developmental life span and be supported in doing so.

## Health Concepts Taught in Other Disciplines

What if teachers of health identified the content knowledge to be shared and promoted by other disciplines, then stayed focused on skill development in their health classes? I believe health educators need to identify the minimum content that is needed by kids as background knowledge. I would argue that background knowledge in health-related topics and concepts will always add to the depth of knowledge a person has, so it should be obtained in personal reading time, extracurricular experiences, and lessons in other disciplinary classes. Because of the limited time allocated for health education in the school curriculum, health educators now try to teach a limited amount of information, called functional knowledge, and stay focused on teaching the skills (and skill sets) needed for the practice of healthful behaviors.

For example, if you want to ensure that students can demonstrate adequate self-care in regard to disease prevention, have students practice hand-washing techniques in health class and help them understand the key questions about that health behavior. You might ask the following:

- What is hand washing?
- Why is it important?
- To what extent should hand washing be practiced in different contexts?
- What adaptations make sense to know and do in new contexts or situations?
- When should you practice hand washing?
- With whom should you practice hand washing?
- Where should hand washing be done?

These question cues use the five Ws of historical thinking to help quantify a habit of health.

It is very important that health educators know how the human story fits into the story of science, social studies, language arts, mathematics, physical education, art, and music. If health education is to have any influence on the health and well-being of students, we must know how the human being gains access to health information through the human senses and then interprets the sensory-motor patterns into cognitive-behavioral patterns of action. Since it is the human being who learns the basic facts, concepts, and theories of the disciplines, we must be able to support all learners so they are healthy and ready to learn. This fundamental premise makes health education essential for all learning.

## Building an Infrastructure for Health Education

Education and health professionals should use the four Ts to build an infrastructure for health education in the school community. The underlying assumption or argument for this infrastructure is that health is foundational to academic achievement.

When writing grants, making programmatic or curricular decisions, and advocating for the health and well-being of children and youth, be sure to build your rationale on one or more of these factors: time, teach, technique, and team.

### Time
Make time for health-related programming

- before school,
- during school, and
- after school.

### Teach

- Teach kids more health education skills every year in health classes.
- Teach kids more health concepts in other disciplinary classes.
- Teach kids health-related life skills in advisory periods.

### Techniques

- Use evidence-based instructional strategies (EBIS), as outlined in chapter 6.
- Use multiple intelligences as a pedagogical language of elements to inform the design of health lessons, as explained in this chapter.

### Team

- Team with health and education professionals to improve the health status of children and youth through the coordinated school health program (CSHP) model, which bridges education, services, and environmental supports for learning.
- Team with all eight academic disciplines to teach health-related concepts through a transdisciplinary curricular approach.

## Need for Professional Teaming in Education and Health

Thus far, I have mentioned several different professionals with design experience (e.g., architects, engineers, landscape designers, interior designers, and teachers). In the construction field, a general contractor coordinates all the different design specialists if the client wishes to hire one. However, the client can also work directly with each design specialist as long as he has the time and expertise to do so.

A general construction contractor welcomes the extra money to do coordination (management) work for a client, much as a curriculum coordinator in a school would coordinate teachers to implement different curricula in social studies, language arts, math, science, or other subjects. Keep in mind that curricula have design elements that are shared between disciplines, but novice teachers may not notice these patterns initially. When teachers have worked with different curricula and programs long enough, common patterns may surface for ease in implementation and integration. Instead of each teacher having to uncover these useful patterns on his or her own, a curriculum coordinator may be able to facilitate knowledge sharing to benefit more teachers and other professionals in the school community (e.g., central administration, school board members, local organizations, and funding agencies).

Unfortunately, not many schools can afford a curriculum coordinator for all academic subjects, so teachers are left to do their own coordinating work within and across grade levels, including how a school articulates with another school in the same district. As one might assume, some teachers are better at this coordinating work than others. When teachers are responsible for implementing many different curricula and programs adopted by the district, they should know what to look for within and between programs.

In health education, teachers have another layer of coordination that goes beyond curriculum implementation in their classrooms. Teachers must also coordinate some of their workday with parents, counselors, nurses, food service employees, psychologists, social workers, special educators, and others, depending on the needs of individual students.

A coordinated school health program model is a multidisciplinary teaming approach for improving the health status of children and youth as advocated by the U.S. Centers for Disease Control and Prevention (2007a). A school district forms a school health advisory council or a health coordinating council (HCC) to bring these key professionals together on a monthly basis to discuss health-related issues and programs. Overall, an HCC provides a needed infrastructure for keeping the focus on a health-promoting school community. Although an HCC focuses on coordination between education and health professionals from the school community, the districts with the most success hire a wellness coordinator who runs the meetings and coordinates prevention and intervention programs.

In my experience with implementing an HCC in a local school district, I have found there needs to be an equal representation of teachers and health professionals from different schools within the district in order to maximize communication, collaboration, and coordination efforts. As a member of an HCC, teachers are responsible for preK-12 prevention initiatives, whereas health professionals are responsible for preK-12 intervention services and supports. In reality, these distinctions are somewhat blurred during the council meetings because everyone must help healthy and unhealthy children equally. However, it is much more effective to focus on and promote an assets-based model for health promotion and disease prevention than a deficit model. Without dedicated time in the academic day for health instruction that focuses on personal skill development of children and youth, an HCC will find itself focused more often on problems and deficits rather than the promotion of health and wellness. Therefore, a comprehensive preK-12 health education curriculum becomes the centerpiece of a successful HCC.

In conclusion, when we educate for health, the curriculum of life focuses on people who need to practice and promote the habits of health and habits of mind on a daily basis. By recognizing a variety of ways to communicate, collaborate, and coordinate, we help to build an infrastructure for health education with our action potentials, action plans, and action research focused on *prevention*.

## CHAPTER FEATURES

### Principles of Practice

• There are six language elements for promoting human health and well-being: words, pictures, numbers, body language, rhythms, and environmental cues. As your own learning increases in sophistication, you will be able to help others uncover and gain access to these multiple ways to educate for health. The key is to use your cognitions to recognize the hidden elements of language so you can design different ways to educate for health (and give young people access to a higher quality of life).

• Multiple intelligences theory can be investigated by looking for various signs, symbols, and patterns across eight different ways of knowing, including the interpersonal and intrapersonal intelligences. A professional who educates for health will use signs, symbols, and patterns as elements for design when planning and implementing health education lessons for individuals and groups. Signs, symbols, and patterns can also be called semiotics.

• Because multiple intelligences theory focuses on problem solving and crafting (designing) products that are valued in one or more cultures, a professional who educates for health will help learners use a variety of language elements (e.g., words, pictures, numbers, rhythms, body language, and environmental cues) to communicate as human beings. These language elements form a subtext to help us to build our understanding and meaning making about topics, concepts, and skills in health education and other disciplines.

• Topics, concepts, and skills serve as a metalanguage, i.e., a common text, when designing lessons for eight academic disciplines, including health education. Topics and concepts are declarative knowledge elements *to know* and skills are procedural knowledge elements *to do*. When educating for health, we design lessons using habits of health and habits of mind. Health-related skills (e.g., decision making, goal setting, communication, stress management, and conflict management) are practiced as habits of mind when educating for health. This curricular distinction allows us to promote cognitive-behavioral outcomes in health education. Habits of health (or health behaviors) often gain in sophistication and intention when integrated and practiced with habits of mind. Children and youth are usually developmental novices in the coordination of their habits of health and habits of mind. Indeed, cognitive-behavioral outcomes in health become a lifelong quest to a higher quality of life.

• When educating for health, we can design interdisciplinary lessons around concepts and skills. Preferences to use transdisciplinary concepts, e.g., change, time, structure, balance, movement, boundaries, cycle, and relationship, across the curriculum in all eight academic disciplines will help to build content knowledge (and ultimately, student background knowledge). This requires that all educators use examples from many different disciplines, including health education. When there are examples about what human beings know and do, including the structure and function of the human body and brain, then there is a greater potential to educate for health across the curriculum. Although the skills of communication, decision making, goal setting, stress management, and conflict management can be found across the academic curriculum in different ways and forms, the health curriculum focuses on how children and youth practice these personal and social skills as daily habits of mind. Therefore, when educating for health, skill development becomes the cognitive centerpiece for our healthy behaviors and must be explicitly taught to young people in our schools, homes, and communities.

• There are universal elements used for communication that form integrative designs and patterns for life. In a way, life is the text when educating for health. These universal elements are used to promote human health and well-being because they help us to communicate and construct meaning about people, places, and things in the world. As your own learning transformation occurs, you will be able to help others gain access to the incredible potential of words, pictures, numbers, body language, rhythms, and environmental cues in designing and interpreting their human story.

• Cognitive psychologists divide knowledge into three types: (1) declarative knowledge, which includes facts, topics, concepts, generalizations, principles, models, and theories; (2) procedural knowledge, which includes skills, strategies, techniques, methods, procedures, and processes; and (3) contextual knowledge, which is based on situational cues of time, space, and place with people and pedagogies. The ways that you use these three types of knowledge in designing health lessons becomes an integrative pattern in educating for health. Basically, you need to weave a story with the elements of topics, concepts, and skills for health education. When you structure your lesson using a lesson plan, students will function or respond based on your plan. The biggest lesson to learn is how to structure a people-centered curriculum in health education (e.g., skill development) rather than an object-centered curriculum (e.g., drugs, toothbrushes, food). This helps young people use the objects for personal reasons and begin to explore the journey to cognitive-behavioral patterns of human health and well-being.

• Novice professionals know one representation of knowledge; expert professionals know multiple representations of knowledge.

• Integrative patterns in educating for health can emerge as you recognize multiple signs, symbols, and patterns as elements of design when communicating health-related messages, lessons, and curricula.

- Habits of mind and habits of health integrate constructivist and behaviorist theories, respectively, when educating for health. Habits of mind and habits of health help you to structure a concise curriculum when educating for health so that your learners will function as healthy human beings on a daily basis. The goal of habits of mind and habits of health is to achieve a higher quality of life through cognitive–behavioral actions of well-being. The use of hands as symbols helps us to make a difference in educating for health.

## Teacher Voices

An early childhood major reflects on a two-week field experience in an elementary school classroom.

Last semester I was placed in an elementary classroom in [a local school] for field experience. I was at the school all day for two straight weeks. During my experience there I did not see much time devoted to health education. Once a week a teacher would rotate through the first grade classroom and teach the kids about safety for 30 minutes. That was all that I saw during my stay there. It is very important that children are taught health habits from the time they are very young. We should be showing the children that health education is important and should be taken seriously. If we are only devoting 30 minutes once a week to health education, what message are we sending the children? I would have liked to have seen more time spent on teaching health as well as health concepts integrated into other disciplines.

*Hope Maglich, Miami University alumna in early childhood education, 2007*

## Seeds of Growth:
## Signs, Symbols, and Patterns of Living and Learning

1. In your learning journal, write or draw responses for each of these language forms to describe your identity:

- What are some words that describe you as a human being?
- What are some numbers that are part of your identity?
- What are some pictures or images of you as a human being?
- What are some ways you move and express yourself through your body language?
- What are some rhythms or sounds that describe you as a human being?
- What are some environmental cues that grab your attention in positive and negative ways as a human being?

2.   In your learning journal, write a song or make a poster that depicts how the "spaces in between" your life have led you to wellness or illness. Nepo states: "Everything is changing and connected. And our call is to enter a dance with the things and forces of this world, not just deflecting what comes at us. For often, the things we need to learn are in the spaces in between" (Nepo, 2005, p. 83).

## Web Links for Living and Learning

Visit the Web sites for the public health campaigns listed in table 4.5 to find health-related information. Determine which habit of health is being promoted for each campaign that targets a specific population of people. After browsing and learning about a campaign in detail, see if you can also find one or more habits of mind being encouraged, so you can use the campaign to help young people develop their skills. To determine the effectiveness of the public health campaign from a communication perspective, please use the checklists in figure 4.3.

Table 4.5   **Public Health Campaigns**

| Title of health campaign | Target population | Web site | Media message |
|---|---|---|---|
| Tobacco vs. Kids: Where America Draws the Line | Children and adolescents | www.tobacco freekids.org | Promote anti-tobacco ads that directly affect children. |
| Powerful Bones. Powerful Girls. | Girls and tweens | www.cdc.gov/ powerfulbones | By participating in weight-bearing activities throughout life, girls can keep their bones strong and prevent bone loss. |
| Car and Home: Smoke Free Zone | People who are smokers | www.smoke freezone.org | Environmental tobacco smoke affects not only your health but also the health of your children. |
| Get Educated, Get Involved | Children and adolescents | www.redcross. org/services/ youth/izone | "Learning about the Red Cross can be fun and easy for young children." |

| Title of health campaign | Target population | Web site | Media message |
|---|---|---|---|
| Fight BAC! Keep Food Safe From Bacteria | All ages | www.fightbac.org | "Fight BAC! Practice safe food handling: Clean, Separate, Cook, Chill." |
| Above the Influence | Adolescents | www.abovetheinfluence.com | "'Be yourself' instead of giving into these pressures." |
| Parents. The Anti-Drug. | Parents | www.theantidrug.com | "Promote parental or caregiver influence in teenagers' lives in a way that ultimately reduces, eliminates, and prevents their drug use." |
| Partnership for a Drug-Free America | Adolescents and their parents | www.drugfree.org | "Drug and substance abuse don't discriminate." |
| Kids Help Line | Ages 5-25 | www.kidshelpline.com | There's always an answer: Seek help. |

## I. Subtext of Human Senses

Please use a check mark to indicate how much your human senses were used when accessing information from the Web site.

| Human senses | Evocative 2 | Enough 1 | Missing 0 |
|---|---|---|---|
| Sight | | | |
| Sound | | | |
| Smell | | | |
| Taste | | | |
| Touch | | | |

Total score = _____ (10 possible points)

**Figure 4.3** Use this form for each Web site visited.

From *Educating for Health: A Reflective Approach to PreK-8 Pedagogy,* by Valerie A. Ubbes, 2008, Champaign, IL: Human Kinetics.

*(continued)*

## II. Subtext of Language Elements

Please use a check mark to indicate which language elements (see page 101) you experienced on the Web site.

| | Objective rating | |
|---|---|---|
| *Signs, symbols, and patterns of language* | Yes = 1 | No = 0 |
| V/L: letters and words as written text and spoken language | | |
| V/S: colors, shapes, images, pictures, icons, graphics, light | | |
| L/M: numbers, sequences, and reasoning | | |
| B/K: kinesthetic, nonverbal body language and expressions, human senses | | |
| M/R: rhythm, music, sound | | |
| N/E: environmental cues from the natural world of plants, animals, and humans | | |

Total score = _____ (6 possible points)

## III. Educational Formats and Communication Channels

Circle the educational *formats* and communication *channels* used to educate for health on the Web site.

| Educational formats | Communication channels |
|---|---|
| Posters, pamphlets, brochures, public service announcements, PowerPoint®, videos, DVDs, Web sites, CD-ROMs, magazines, journals, art, books (e.g., picture narrative, information expository, text), songs, music, dance, nature, newspapers | Interpersonal, radio, television, phone Where? On location: _____ Or setting: _____ |

**Figure 4.3** *(continued)*

### Books for Living and Learning

Read *When Cody Became a Mouse Potato* (Nygard & Koonce, 2002). Look for the multiple ways the book compares and contrasts humans and animals and makes analogies to different disciplinary stories. At the end of the book, there are learning links to the eight multiple intelligences. After what you have learned about the signs, symbols, and patterns of different languages in this chapter, you can now see how teachers develop assignments for a well-balanced lifestyle.

# 5

# Ways to Structure Stories: Personal and Professional Frameworks

It is not by accident that Native American medicine men put these questions to the sick who are brought to them: When was the last time you sang? When was the last time you danced? When was the last time you told your story? When was the last time you listened to stories of others? It has always been clear that the life of our expression and the life of our stories are connected to our health.

© by Mark Nepo, *The Exquisite Risk: Daring to Live an Authentic Life*, 2005

Hanley (2004) offers the following comment about stories:

> Once upon a time there was the word. As the word took form it became story. Stories told us who we were, who we were not, what we remembered, and what we dreamed. They made us wonder. Sometimes the story was transformative; it made us see the world in different ways, and, sometimes, from different perspectives. The story took on many forms. Some stories, like science and math, are about the natural world; some, like literature, arts, and politics, are stories about human experience. Some stories, like social theory, help us to interpret other stories. On a more fundamental level, all our stories are about natural and social experience because humans are of both. (p. 21)

Geertz (1973) talks about the social web of meaning as "webs of significance that man himself has spun" (p. 5). Hanley (2004) suggests that "web is an informative metaphor, which implies the multiple interconnections of meaning in culture. Significance can mean signs and symbols, and it is also a synonym for worth and meaning" (p. 22). Hanley continues:

> Teachers are storytellers and the stories they tell are structured from the conflicts of culture and formed into curricula. . . . Pedagogy is the performance of curriculum between teacher and student. Like curriculum, pedagogy has an aesthetic. When a teacher and learner connect, create meaning, and form new knowledge, what can be more beautiful than that? The give and take of teachers and learners, like dance, is about the mutual communication of meaning, on so much more than a verbal surface. (pp. 22-23)

Irwin (2004) highlights quilts as metaphors of connection and community. Kind (2004) suggests that "when only one story is told, that of comfort and connection, it misses the actual cutting, opening, and wounding that are fundamental to textile process" (p. 49). Kind continues: "Stitch. Cut. Knit together. Unravel. Textiles take shape as processes of constructing and undoing; meaning and opening; seaming and cutting. . . . I see pedagogy and the text of curriculum take shape as an artistic, textured, textile text" (p. 51).

## Ways to Structure Stories

Each person learns many stories throughout life, and it is through these stories—some factual and others fictional—that one gains access to a personal, private, and eventually professional philosophy. Some questions guide the important task before you: Will you include the story of health in your classroom? How will you tell the stories of health and education? How will you help children and youth gain access to their own personal stories through a wellness or illness framework? How much time and attention will you give health-related topics, concepts, and skills in your curriculum? What is the rationale for teaching health education as a focused component of the academic curriculum *and* as conceptual content for other disciplinary stories? To what extent will kids get time to solve their own health issues and problems in your class? To what extent will kids be co-creators of health lessons so they can construct personal meaning about healthy and harmful patterns in their lives with your guiding support? What health-related messages and behaviors will you model and advance as part of your teaching philosophy? And the list goes on.

Over the years, you have used communication as an important way of forming your identity. Educational theorists encourage you to use multiple forms of literacy (e.g., reading, writing, speaking), including multiple intelligences, to reach and teach people about education. Regarding the latter, I hope this text has helped you learn how to access information through multiple language elements (e.g., words, pictures, numbers, body language, rhythms, and environmental cues) so you will interpret the patterns and symbol systems for effective instructional design. Education is certainly grounded in effective communication, and you must be skilled in multiple language forms in order to model what you will expect from your learners.

As we explore the multiple story lines of this text, please appreciate the myriad choices you have in crafting and integrating your story about education *and* health. *Integration* comes from the Latin word *integer*, meaning whole. Hence, integration means to bring your stories together into a whole. So far, these stories have been evolving: personal and professional stories, education and health stories, your stories and your students' stories, and habits of health and habits of mind. In this section, we look at picture book narrative stories and informational expository text, then at story and theory.

## Use of Children's Literature

I believe we should include informational books (expository text) in tandem with picture books (narrative stories) to give children and youth greater access to information about health and life. Picture books and informational texts are an excellent way to educate for health. The elements of narrative picture books are character, setting, sequence of events, plot, problem, and resolution. Fisher and Medvic (2003) suggest that young people can learn how to change the elements of a story by describing what might have happened if a major event had occurred earlier, later, or not at all. The elements of informational texts are description, sequence, compare and contrast, cause and effect, problem, and solution. When informational texts are used for health education, you establish the supports for authentic and often realistic uses of information.

In a study of first-grade classrooms, Duke (2000) found that students spent only 3.6 minutes each day interacting with informational text. When using informational texts in health education, students can practice the integrated communication processes of reading, writing, talking, and listening. For example, students can read about the human body, then write a letter asking questions of a local doctor, dentist, chiropractor, or school nurse. Students can also be asked to prepare a brochure for a peer about how to take care of a human sense, body part, or body system. Students are often eager to craft a poster with a health-related message or to make a leaflet with the sequential steps for flossing teeth, preparing a healthful snack, or crossing the street safely. These informational approaches help students communicate and construct meaning for their personal health.

Informational approaches for increasing health communication and literacy can foster students' active engagement with written texts and provoke important retellings that foster verbal and nonverbal communication skills. If the retellings are stories about their personal health, children can practice active listening skills in the context of building relationships with the information and each other.

## Differences Between the Frameworks of Story and Theory

In this section, we move into the comparison between story and theory. As professionals, personal stories are important, but it is now time to understand and appreciate the value of theory, a professional form of story. In education, we often focus on the concept pairs of theory and practice. In this context, practice becomes a form of personal story. According to Sanchez (1994), "Theory and practice, if they are to inform each other meaningfully, must operate in a constant state of mutually transformative flux" (p. 22).

In his text *Constructing Knowledges*, Dobrin (1997) makes the following statement:

> Etymologically, theory is derived from the Latin *theoria* and the Greek *theros*, both of which refer to the "spectator," which is closely related to "speculum." *Theory* is also derived from or related to *theasthai*, "to observe or view," and *theōrin*, "to consider." The work itself suggests an empirical grounding: that a theory is derived from direct observation. Thus, someone who theorizes is a kind of "spectator," closely "observing" some reality and "mirroring" (as a speculum, or mirror, does) the observed phenomenon in pre-

cise descriptions on its nature. The theorist then "considers" or "speculates" on the nature of the phenomenon in order to arrive at generalizable statements, or universal truths, about how all members of the class to which the observed phenomenon belongs work. (pp. 7-8)

Dobrin (1997) suggests that the real value of theory is the ability of experts to adapt and change theory based on new experiences and observations. "Because of their evolutionary quality, theories are not usually seen in terms of *true* or *false*; rather, new theories are seen as more adequate or more useful explanations of phenomena for which past theories could not account. Theory leaves room for revision; universal explanations can be rethought" (p. 9).

Thus far, we have explored the role of three educational theories in health education: learning styles theory in chapter 2, constructivist theory in chapter 3, and multiple intelligences theory in chapter 4. This chapter makes a case for comparing story and theory.

## Professional Stories of Health Education

I have tried to make this book a story of teaching *and* learning about health. Rather than expecting you to understand all the health-related issues of children and youth, I chose to focus on the integrative patterns of the five senses, wellness, habits of health, and habits of mind as the foundational content for your role as a teacher. With experience, you will know how to design health-related lessons and units that are developmentally appropriate, culturally sensitive, body–brain compatible, and health enhancing. Your lessons and units will be aligned to local, state, and national standards for health education. This text also advocates for your personal health and wellness so that you can effectively manage the changes in your day.

As you prepare to educate for health, the following questions will help frame your professional practice:

- How can you support children and youth to integrate and practice their habits of health and habits of mind so that they can have a healthy quality of life?

- How does your integrated knowledge of education and health theories help children and youth gain access and competence to use valid health information, products, and services?

- How does your philosophy of "who you are and what you know" interact with your pedagogy of "what you do with who you know" so that your personal stories and professional theories have integrity in health education?

# My Professional Philosophy

In 2006, I was invited to speak about one of the five philosophical perspectives in health education, as a member on a national panel. Backed by a paper outlining constructivist theory for health education (Ubbes, Black, & Ausherman, 1999), I presented my rationale for a cognitive philosophy of health education. As I listened to other members of the panel, I found myself respectfully identifying with each of their philosophical perspectives as well. When professionals gather at conferences, there are often overlapping nuances in the shared information. I could see how my interest in cognitive theories formed a larger story informed by the other four perspectives.

When professionals tell the stories and hypotheses of their disciplines, they use quantitative and qualitative data to document their findings. Research is an ongoing process of re-searching the smaller stories that emerge from well-defined studies. Each story helps tell the larger story of the discipline. Sometimes the findings are similar, and sometimes the findings are different. But the purpose of the ongoing research is to seek patterns and trends in the information over time.

My presentation highlighted the cognitive perspective of health education because of my commitment to thinking processes and the role of inquiry in health education—especially body–mind connections. I stated then, as I do now, that health education needs to build a stronger case for sensory-motor and cognitive-behavioral theories. These approaches help define how information is processed and acted on through prior knowledge, motivations, and intentions to act. I recognize that people also learn how to learn in the context of sociocultural and environmental cues.

I am convinced of the need for age-appropriate developmental theories that move human beings into more sophisticated patterns of solving problems and crafting products and performances. The discipline of health education is rich with different theories to explain health behaviors, but thus far little attention has been focused on information processing. By mapping three educational theories (constructivist theory, learning styles theory, and multiple intelligences theory) into health education, I hope to deepen our understanding of how learners differentiate their responses to health-related messages, including the changing effects of sociocultural and environmental cues in educating for health. Ultimately, it is important to know if these theories help explain how people gain access to health-related information through their sensory-motor responses to the environment, supported by how they cognitively access information through learning styles and multiple intelligences when constructing meaning (and ultimately actions) for health. In most cases, a personal story gains new meaning when told in community, owing to the power and influence of significant others in our lives.

# My Personal Philosophy

My professional story is supported by personal stories that highlight the role of community partnerships in youth development. I grew up in the German Turner organization, whose motto is "a sound mind in a sound body." The Turner movement, begun in Germany in 1811, stresses physical fitness and German culture. German immigrants brought the movement to the United States in the 1840s and in 1850 established a national Turner association that is today known as the American Turners. For most of my formative years, I practiced gymnastics and other forms of physical activity in the context of a sociocultural environment. "A sound mind *in* a sound body" told me then (as it does now) that inside my body I have a sound mind to care for and support with the physical structure of my human form. In this context, *sound* means without defect or damage as well as thorough and complete. As a young person, "a sound mind in a sound body" made sense and gave focus to my life.

If I were to pursue a historical study of "a sound mind in a sound body," I would be assuming the role of a philosopher, who often problematizes ideas to discuss them. In this case, the phrase can be discussed as a Cartesian debate of dualism. But as a youth and even as a young adult, I knew nothing about this academic discussion. I know that as a young person, I found comfort and even guidance in the language of body and mind; I formed a strong identity through my actions in physical activity and sport by participating with my brothers, sisters, and friends in many formal and informal activities in the sociocultural venue of the American Turner Club.

In my formative years, I was also a Girl Scout and the secretary of our local 4-H Cooperative Extension organization. Through the latter, I learned that my head, heart, hands, and health were connected for better living. My developmental years in the YMCA offered a place "to put Christian principles into practice through programs that build healthy spirit, mind and body for all." Today, the motto for the YMCA states, "We build strong kids, strong families, strong communities" through the values of faith, caring, honesty, respect, and responsibility.

In an academic sense, these developmental experiences were structured events that molded and shaped me to live a healthy life within a group of people with a common membership. I am very thankful for the community organizations that laid my philosophy for health and wellness, especially since I did not have formal health education until ninth grade in public school (for only one semester!) and only one course in college. It wasn't until my doctoral studies in health education that I understood what represented health education and what didn't. During that time, I read the peer-reviewed professional journals of health education, along with academic books, which influenced my personal story with professional theories about health education.

So what generalizations or "take-home" messages did I derive from health education experiences as a youth and later as an adult? In some ways then and without question now, I am able to appreciate the multiplicity of perspectives that different people believe in and adopt through their decisions to act. I am thankful for the theme of well-being as a major subtext in my life from the age of three when I began gymnastics at the Turner Club—right through to the YMCA membership that my family currently holds. These guiding principles and mottos of organizations in my life did inform me but did not dictate or demand that I put out or get out. The freedom to come and go with the choice to participate was guided by my parents and youth leaders, who orchestrated the details and logistics of schedules, finances, and commitments of time and energy to these daily experiences.

As a health educator in my adult years, I believe it is critical to have these community partnerships available to children, youth, and their families during their formative years. The interconnections that young people can make between home, community organizations, and schools are essential in building a strong infrastructure for health promotion and disease prevention in their lives. This infrastructure is very much a hidden and transparent web of interconnectivity (or not) in a child's life. How caring adults weave that web can sustain a young child's life in very concrete ways.

In preK-12 health education, the guiding framework of curriculum standards directs professionals who will educate for health. The National Health Education Standards (Joint Committee on NHES, 2007) highlight the skill set that young people need to practice, which I have named habits of mind (e.g., decision making, goal setting, communication, stress management, and conflict resolution). To help young people practice these skills requires bridging experiences to habits of health that are reinforced in school, at home, and in the community. As adults, we need to plan for these bridging experiences even though children and youth are limited by concrete thinking in the here and now. By viewing health education as a lifelong connected experience, you may be more willing to structure skill-based lessons that function as a bridge between school, home, and community partnerships. Such partnerships can weave a supportive infrastructure of health and wellness as a safety net for life.

## Philosophy of How to Educate for Health

It is my experience that many people do not know their bodies very well. Some people recognize their bodies only when they are ill. Many people have learned to ignore stomach pains, headaches, and the need for sleep. People use clothing, piercings, jewelry, and tattoos to decorate their outside identities, but many do not understand their bodies below the surface. Few express awe and wonder about the design of the human form. When we educate for health, we need thoughtful learning processes that give people access to their internal bodies and minds instead of being distracted by the external outward view of cosmetics and ways to mask some of our aches and pains.

I believe we can do a better job of teaching people how to consciously connect to their physical being, social being, intellectual being, spiritual being, and emotional being by focusing on body language and its cues (e.g., thirst, temperature, fatigue). Such conscious awareness begins as sensory messages in the form of sight, sound, smell, taste, and touch but grows to a deeper appreciation of how the brain communicates its findings back to the individual. In all our human senses, the external body organ or receptor does a fine job of collecting the sensory information, but until our minds masterfully interpret the data, we don't have the ability to see, hear, smell, taste, or touch. The body and brain work together to learn and adapt to changing environments and experiences.

We need to consciously pay attention to environmental cues that influence our human senses and cognitive pathways. Indeed, there is a difference between hearing and listening; sight and seeing; touch and feeling. Young people often copy and mimic the health actions of others thanks to mirror neurons and their networks that connect to the cerebellum, the brain structure that coordinates muscular movements. Ramachandran and Oberman (2006) report that mirror neurons are also located in other brain structures, such as the insula and the anterior cingulate cortex, which may play a role in emotional responses that show empathy. Mirror neurons are also important for enabling "humans to see themselves as others see them, which may be an essential ability for self-awareness and introspection" (p. 65).

My own interest in health education is focused on how people gain access to valid and reliable health information during their formative years and how they interpret and use different forms of information to learn about themselves, others, and the world around them. Much of the environmental information that enters our senses comes in the form of light waves and sound waves, as repeating rhythmical patterns. As you learned in chapter 2 in the discussion on learning styles, individuals do vary in their processing of information and to what extent they attend to and respond consciously to these data, including whether they interpret information objectively or subjectively.

When educating for health, we can help learners attend to the role of their human senses in processing information. I believe that those professionals who delight in educating for health cannot ignore the benefits of this approach in connecting learning to the human mind and body. To promote our human response to information as either background data to be ignored or as conscious cues to action may be the future of health promotion.

## Multiple Professional Perspectives in Health

As I see it, the current investigations in health-related professions involve four perspectives: health education (i.e., how people learn about health), health sciences (i.e., how the basic sciences of the human body are affected by health and disease), health behavior (i.e., how behavioral outcomes are associated with mortality, morbidity, and longevity), and health communication (i.e., how different communication elements affect the health-related choices of humans in their environments). These four perspectives, shown in figure 5.1 as a backdrop to the ecological model (figure 2.1), are ways that people in health-related professions have interpreted the field. These professional interpretations are analogous to someone in the music profession who has an interest in telling and

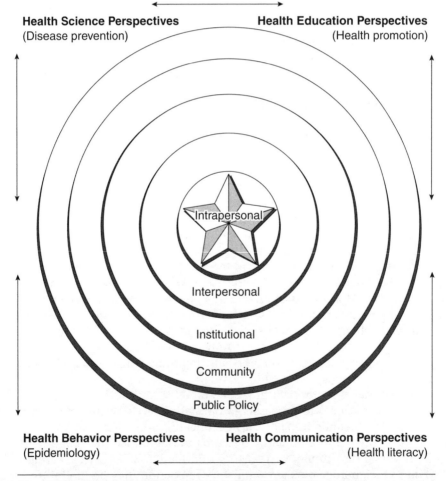

**Health Science Perspectives**
(Disease prevention)

**Health Education Perspectives**
(Health promotion)

Intrapersonal

Interpersonal

Institutional

Community

Public Policy

**Health Behavior Perspectives**
(Epidemiology)

**Health Communication Perspectives**
(Health literacy)

**Figure 5.1** Multiple health perspectives inform the ecological model.

retelling the stories of music as jazz, country western, baroque, hip-hop, or any of the other musical genres.

Genres are ways that professionals in a discipline (e.g., science) or a domain (e.g., photography) have interpreted and crafted new stories or findings. These tellings and retellings are interpretations of one perspective in a world of multiple interpretations. Disciplinary perspectives in health education are constantly changing and being guided by professionals who help define them.

As a profession continues to refine its models and theories, different perspectives emerge as a way to tell the stories of the disciplines. Such thematic stories are shared in academic books like this one to help young professionals recognize the trends in the field. When you educate for health, you will never know if you will play a role in influencing the future career of your students. Because health education is underrepresented in the preK-12 experience, many young people do not consider health-related careers until late in their academic preparation. Unfortunately, I did not hear enough stories of health in my preK-16 development. I entered the profession of health education after my second year of doctoral studies at the age of 28. I found health education; it didn't find me. My personal story emerged at the crossroads of the health professions that I have been investigating for the last two decades.

Now I would like to show you how story and theory can be "problematized." As you read what Postman writes below about bias in education, think about the four perspectives that I have outlined for you in figure 5.1.

Postman (1995) shares the following insights about how bias plays a role in education:

> Suppose teachers made it clear that all the materials introduced in class were not to be regarded as authoritative and final but, in fact, as problematic—textbooks, for example. . . . We would start with the premise that a textbook is a particular person's attempt to explain something to us, and thereby tell us the truth of some matter. But we would know that this person could not be telling us the whole truth. Because no one can. We would know that this person has certain prejudices and biases. Because everyone has. We would know that this person must have included some disputable facts, shaky opinions, and faulty conclusions. Thus, we have good reason to use this person's textbook as an object of inquiry. What might have been left out? What are the prejudices? What are the disputable facts, opinions, and conclusions? How would we proceed to make such an inquiry? Where would we go to check facts? What is a "fact," anyway? How would we proceed in uncovering prejudice? On what basis would we judge a conclusion unjustifiable? (p. 126)

By reading peer-reviewed professional journals and books and attending professional conferences, you will gain more insights into the diverse interpretations that exist in the field of health. As you craft your professional story and weave your personal and professional stories together in a context unique for you, you will write your own story about educating for health. You could choose to keep this story to yourself, but it is more collegial to share what you know with other professionals. In the process of sharing your ideas in a community of learners, you will learn more about who you are as a professional, including new ways to refine and extend your story about life and learning.

## My Interpretation of the Ecological Model

As a consistent reader of education and health literature, I am able to see how the two fields are alike and different in their approaches to life issues, problems, and events. Since I have memberships in both education and health organizations, I have access to a growing literature through journal articles and books in those fields. I also try to read outside my field, in neuroscience, because I find great interest in how the brain works and how it functions. I deeply appreciate how my brain is responsible for my quality of life, providing an aesthetic experience in interpreting the beauty of a flower and the complexities of a genome pattern.

I am now going to demonstrate how I integrate a public health model and an educational theory to form the contextual model of human expertise. Empirical studies and scholarly discourse about my model will need to occur before it can be accepted as a theoretical model for health education.

To begin with, the intrapersonal and interpersonal levels of the ecological model are not closed systems. In figure 5.2, I have enlarged the core of the ecological model to show how these levels interact. Since this text focuses heavily on your identity development as the core of your personal and professional stories, it may be useful to study the complexities of this model at its core.

First, notice that access between the intrapersonal and interpersonal levels occurs by a bridge on the right side of the figure. The bridge can be imagined as a pathway all the way through the five levels of the ecological model, but it is especially important at these two levels because each person needs access to other people in the world. The star at the core reminds us that the human senses model is inherent in each individual who can perceive other people through human interaction in a shared place or space. The five human sense organs form sensory pathways into the brain so that seeing, hearing, smelling, tasting, and touching can occur. Without the brain's interpretation of electromagnetic (light) and mechanical (sound and touch) signals entering the human nervous

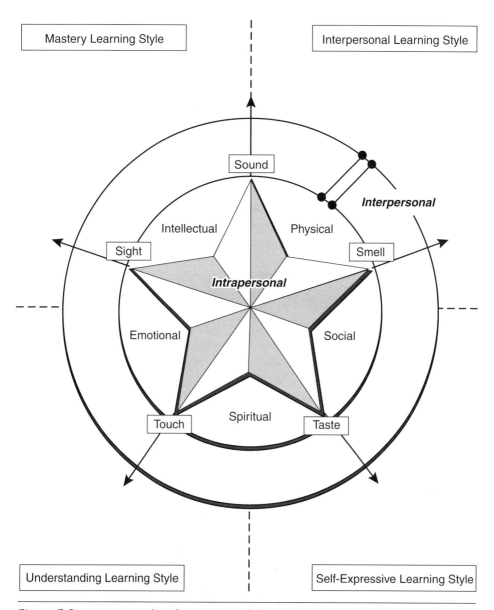

**Figure 5.2**  Intrapersonal and interpersonal levels of influence are linked by learning styles.

system, there will be no perception. Table 5.1 shows how information signals are used by humans for communication. You can also see how there are intersensory responses (e.g., aural, visual, kinesthetic) from the human senses. In chapter 2, we talked about the two-dimensional aspect

Table 5.1 **Information Signals Used by Humans for Communication**

| Multiple intelligences | Information signals used by humans for communication | Intersensory responses from the human senses | Selected examples of perceptual motor skills |
|---|---|---|---|
| Verbal linguistic | Mechanical sound waves, electromagnetic light waves, electrochemical brain waves | Aural, visual, but can also be kinesthetic for individuals who are blind | Talking, singing |
| Visual spatial | Electromagnetic light waves, electrochemical brain waves | Visual, equilibrium | Seeing, balancing |
| Logical mathematical | Mechanical sound waves, electromagnetic light waves, electrochemical brain waves | Aural, visual, kinesthetic | Counting, sequencing |
| Bodily kinesthetic | Mechanical body pressure, mechanical body position, body temperature, electrochemical brain waves | Gustatory, olfactory, tactile, kinesthetic, visual, aural | Moving with locomotor and non-locomotor skills; moving with manipulative skills |
| Musical rhythmical | Mechanical sound waves, electromagnetic light waves, electrochemical brain waves | Aural, kinesthetic, tactile | Humming, fingering instrument |
| Naturalist environmental | Mechanical sound waves, electromagnetic light waves, air and water pressure, air and water temperature, electrochemical brain waves | Gustatory, olfactory, tactile, kinesthetic, visual, aural | Observing, perceiving, responding |

of each of our basic human senses. Our human senses help us perceive the people, places, and things of the world, so it makes sense that we promote the human senses when we educate for health.

In chapter 2, I also introduced the wellness space of human well-being model, which uses an open pathway between each dimension of health, forming a star pattern at its core (see figure 2.6). These pathways are how individuals at the intrapersonal level of the ecological model access their human senses and have the potential to build a well human being each day. If space and time are lacking in a person's life on any given day, there is limited access to wellness. Over time, one can imagine that a wellness model can become an illness model. For those individuals who are well on a consistent basis and constantly shining from their core beings, the waves of light and sound vibrate outward from the ecological model to different institutions and communities, where they can have a positive influence on other human beings.

The third important aspect of figure 5.2 is the four windows of opportunity, or learning styles, which were also described in chapter 2. The four learning styles, from left to right, then top to bottom, are mastery, interpersonal, understanding, and self-expressive. Although all four learning styles give people different ways to access and learn information, the interpersonal learning style is especially important in this context because it has the same name as the second level of the ecological model. Therefore, I believe that learning styles theory from the education literature and the ecological model from the health literature are well suited for cross-disciplinary connections.

In a literal sense, a person who prefers to access information through human interaction as an interpersonal learner will be quite adept at interpersonal relations in health promotion. However, because an intrapersonal (self) perspective is foundational to the interpersonal (other) level of the ecological model, one must be willing to strike a balance between self-study and people study. In fact, to be effective as a professional who will educate for health, you need adaptability and flexibility in accessing health-related information from all four windows of opportunity, so you can help others get access to what you know.

## Principles of Practice: The Contextual Model of Human Expertise

Figure 5.3 shows a revised ecological model called the contextual model of human expertise. Two distinct changes are seen in the revised ecological model for health promotion. First, a star symbol is officially placed at the core of the intrapersonal level of the model. By now, you know that the star represents the role of the human senses in observing and perceiving the world. The star also symbolizes how an individual becomes enlightened to become a well human being. In the background space behind the star, though not labeled here, a wellness model exists for daily guidance in physical being, social being, emotional being, spiritual being, and intellectual being. As we integrate our human senses and human well-being on a daily basis, we have the opportunity to form a more integral core to our world perspective. Second, the words *public policy* from the fifth level of the ecological model have been replaced by *sources of knowledge*. I spent a great deal of time naming this level and was concerned that the words were too abstract. Then I read that

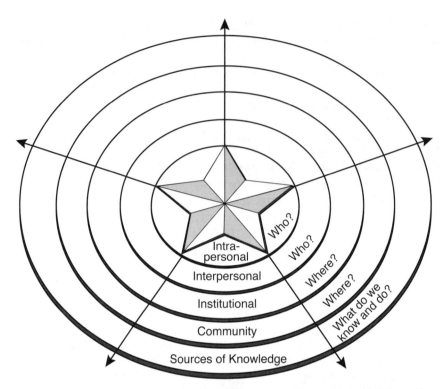

Intra-
personal

Interpersonal

Institutional

Community

Sources of Knowledge

Who?
Who?
Where?
Where?
What do we
know and do?

| Influence | Level of Ecological Model | Perspectives to Consider |
|-----------|---------------------------|--------------------------|
| People | Intrapersonal and interpersonal | Culture, age, race, ethnicity, gender, status |
| Places | Institutions and communities | Setting, place, geographical location |
| Things | Sources of knowledge to use, adapt, or develop | Papers, pamphlets, posters, performances, presentations, professional code of ethics, props, public service announcements, publications, plans, programs, procedures, policies, position statements, principles of practice, pedagogy, people interaction, personal philosophy |

**Figure 5.3** Contextual model of human expertise.

Adapted, by permission, from J.M. Eddy et al., 2002, "Application of an ecological perspective in worksite health promotion: A review," *American Journal of Health Studies* 17(4): 197-202.

a philosophy is a form of inquiry that explores the nature of human knowledge and the sources of knowledge. That last phrase concretized my thinking.

Table 5.2 defines different sources of knowledge that frame the outer level of the contextual model of human expertise. It is contextual because it highlights "what you know and what you do" in a particular context (e.g., institution in a community).

As you move from passive (received) knowledge to active (constructed) knowledge, you learn to *make* meaning. For example, you learn to solve problems and contribute to the world by making health-related props, products, and programs, to name a few. By making (designing) these sources of knowledge, you make a difference in the world. At first, you come to know the many sources of knowledge as a way to promote health; then you learn to make and refine other sources of knowledge for yourself and others.

### Table 5.2   Multiple Sources of Knowledge

| Sources of knowledge *to know* | Sources of knowledge *to make or do* |
|---|---|
| ✔ Papers (e.g., essays, narratives, grant proposals, reports, research) | ✔ Papers (e.g., essays, narratives, grant proposals, reports, research) |
| ✔ Pamphlets, brochures, leaflets | ✔ Pamphlets, brochures, leaflets |
| ✔ Posters | ✔ Posters |
| ✔ Performances and presentations | ✔ Performances and presentations |
| ✔ Professional code of ethics and dispositions | ✔ Professional code of ethics and dispositions |
| ✔ Props and artifacts | ✔ Props and artifacts |
| ✔ Public service announcements and campaigns | ✔ Public service announcements and campaigns |
| ✔ Publications (e.g., print and electronic) | ✔ Publications (e.g., print and electronic) |
| ✔ Plans or models | ✔ Plans or models |
| ✔ Programs and curricula | ✔ Programs and curricula |
| ✔ Procedures and processes | ✔ Procedures and processes |
| ✔ Policies and laws | ✔ Policies and laws |
| ✔ Position statements and letters to editors and boards | ✔ Position statements and letters to editors and boards |
| ✔ Principles of practice and pedagogy | ✔ Principles of practice and pedagogy |
| ✔ People interactions in verbal and nonverbal ways | ✔ People interactions in verbal and nonverbal ways |
| ✔ Personal philosophy and journal reflections | ✔ Personal philosophy and journal reflections |

The sources of knowledge *to know* and the sources of knowledge *to make or do* are the same on both sides of table 5.2. Each of them begins with a letter P to reflect the patterns of expertise that we have when educating for health. You can make multiple representations of knowledge through many interpretive forms. Interpretations are explanations or meanings that you give to an object or a subjective idea from your own perspective. As a professional who will educate for health, you are learning about the many sources of knowledge. You will continue to refine the many sources of knowledge as you promote health for yourself and others in the world. Your expertise will evolve when you modify these knowledge sources to fit a new situation or context. Again, those situations or contexts are the places known as institutions and communities, as shown in figure 5.3. Many of you will educate for health in schools, but some of you will educate for health in community agencies, youth organizations, clinics, and other institutions.

## Human Beings as Human Doings

Neuroscience is clear that all behaviors are mediated by the brain unless we are dealing with a reflex. Therefore, cognition (thought) is an important place to start in understanding health behaviors (i.e., what we do with what we know). Up until now, we have traveled through four chapters: who we are, ways to be, ways to think, and ways to know. This chapter emphasizes what we do with what we know.

In teenage years, poor choices and follow-the-leader mentalities result when young people are influenced by unhealthy role models in different social contexts or in the media. Young people may show irresponsible behaviors because their neural connections between the prefrontal cortex and the cerebellum that are responsible for motor control and physical actions are not fully developed (i.e., myelinated). You can increase neuronal connections to the cerebellum and vice versa by giving your students practice time to learn sensory-motor skills (e.g., stress relaxation exercises) and cognitive-behavioral skills (e.g., refusing a tobacco offer) during your classroom scenarios. When your students "learn to move and move to learn," they increase their intellectual health and physical health.

Moving and doing something with what you know also stimulates the other dimensions of your health. For these reasons, we should educate for health in active ways instead of expecting children to watch simulations or just talk about everything. You should not expect your students to learn how to wash hands, for example, by simply watching a video. They must be cued to action, given feedback on their actual technique, and given the environmental supports to practice this skill in multiple places and contexts. When we educate for health, our students can use their changing stories about life and health as their text. In the next section, we look at how to also use curriculum as the text.

# Curriculum as Text

Curriculum, from the Latin *currere*, to run or chart a course, is the foundation on which all disciplines are built. The curriculum of life is health. In education, there are multiple ways of asking questions about curriculum. Discourses move from left to right in liberal to conservative ideas of voice and choice—even within the democratic principles of freedom. As educators, we must acknowledge how the curriculum may offer an advantage or a disadvantage to certain perspectives and people. What knowledge is of most worth? For whose interests are curriculum decisions determined? Does the curriculum to educate for health give young people voice and choice to access valid and reliable forms of information? Is this information relevant to their lives during their developmental years? Does your professional voice help shape the curriculum for health in different institutions and communities? If educational disciplines are built and rebuilt from the courses of their curricula, we must be willing to hear the smaller stories of each professional within the larger stories of the discipline. When like-minded individuals join to form community support for certain agendas, their actions result in curriculum. Each organization, institution, and group began with one person joining another person in a pattern of activity toward a common goal.

Figure 5.4 shows how professionals who educate for health structure their work as curriculum, instruction, and assessment. Your expertise will improve as you observe and study how these three educational elements are related and function together. Figure 5.5 shows that educational theory and practice continue to change and adapt because of professionals who practice the skills of assessing learners; planning, implementing, and evaluating lessons of the curriculum; coordinating people and services; and acting as resource people through effective communication in multiple forms (e.g., reading, writing, speaking, and listening).

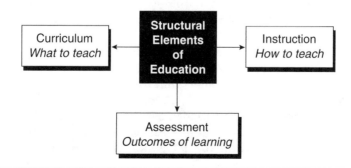

**Figure 5.4** Structural elements of education.

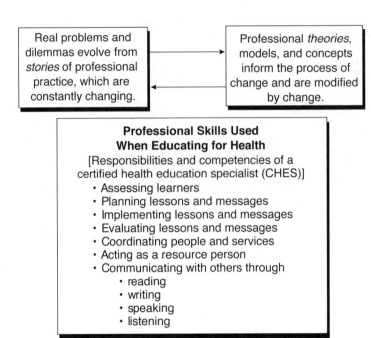

Figure 5.5   The dynamic relationship between stories of professional practice and professional theories.

Our individual beliefs and values feel better in a community, but we cannot be egocentric and ideological to the point of blind faith. In your classroom (and in your school community), you will observe that whenever someone has a voice, there are many others who do not have a voice or choice. The balancing act between individuals and groups determines the balance of power. When power moves beyond assertive acts into aggressive or passive results, the voice of authority is not shared. As adults, each of us can author our own lives and learning. That principle cannot be lost to chance when educating for health. As guardian ad litem for children, you also need to join with other professionals in the school community to link children and youth with programs and services to support their healthy growth and development.

Even though you will focus on your own health and wellness on a daily basis, you must be mindful of moving outward from your core to influence a greater community. This community might be your own classroom of students; your family and friends; a public interest group that is local, regional, or national in scope; or professional causes and organizations. People who are tired and unhealthy cannot perform assertive acts of courage. Only those professionals who are well will have the endurance and insight to move forward with resiliency to serve the greater community of learners while targeting the individual needs of students.

In the next section, we will take a historical look at one of the three structural elements of education: curriculum. Curriculum tells both a story and the theory of a discipline, and is a framework that evolves from instructional design to answer the question "What will learners know and be able to do as a result of the educational journey through the curriculum?" We will address pedagogy—that is, instruction and assessment—in the next chapter.

# Historical and Philosophical Perspectives of Curriculum

In 1918, Franklin Bobbitt published his text *The Curriculum*, which outlined a particular protocol for curriculum development. His administrative procedural approach to the study of curriculum inspired other educators, most notably Ralph Tyler, who published *Basic Principles of Curriculum and Instruction* in 1949. To this day, curriculum scholars refer to Tyler's work as the Tyler rationale, in which curriculum development is a procedural exercise.

Elliot Eisner (2004), a noted curriculum scholar and professor at Stanford University, with joint appointments in the School of Education and School of Art, suggests the following:

> Too much of what we do in school caters to routine. Too much of what we do is mired in tradition and stale habit; too much is formulaic and prescriptive. There is a paucity of genuine invention in education and the concept of artistry might help alleviate the constraints that over formalized and highly-technologized processes sometimes impose. (p. 16)

In the curriculum field, Pinar, Reynolds, Slattery, and Taubman (1995) and Dewey (1934) viewed curriculum as a "verb, growing, creating, and being, instead of a mere noun, a flat thing to be consumed and digested" (Mullen, 2004, p. 32).

Each year as you educate for health, you will learn that your choices in the curriculum are often guided on a macrolevel by guidelines, standards, and policies. You are only one teacher of many who contribute to the decision making, but your voice and choice are important to the whole.

Your balance point between dependent and independent choices will emerge when you respect the interdependency of people who are young and old, novice and expert, and common and diverse as they negotiate their own curriculum of life. Your role as a teacher is to help people solve problems to make the world a better place as they learn to think like historians, scientists, mathematicians, writers, planners, leaders, or any other contributors to society. Each of these professionals will need the discipline to promote a personal health agenda because the curriculum of life is health. So your role in giving people access to their wellness and quality of life is vital. The dependent and independent choices of people who can integrate wellness into their daily lives are, indeed, a transformational part of the school curriculum.

McDermott (2004) reminds us that we can achieve transformative thinking and living by wandering away from the straight and narrow pathways available to us. She claims that "artistic thinkers are wanderers as well, encouraging others to move off narrow and well-tread paths of thinking or seeing the world" (p. 67). She contrasts teaching and learning in the early 20th century as a production model with "clearly defined. . . measurable and predetermined tasks which lead the process simply from A to B, with little room for deviation, or wandering" with teaching and learning as a creative model that allows one "to think, see, and do curriculum, as an aesthetic text with style" (p. 68).

McDermott speaks about the power of curriculum as "re-imagine[d] through the visions of an artist, a curriculum in which we, as educators, and our students have the right to choose. In our wanderings we transgress off the path mandated by a fixed one-size-fits-all model of curriculum" (p. 69).

Flinders (2004) also writes about the synergy between curriculum and pedagogy as inspired by the arts:

> With respect to art in general, we often associate an aesthetic experience with works that present multiple layers of meaning. In drama, music, poetry and the like, we readily speak of sub-texts, foreshadowing, deconstructed meanings, symbolism, allusions, understatement, connotations, irony, metaphors, allegories, and themes. This lexicon implies that one purpose of art is to take us behind the scenes of an experience or beneath the surface of what we would otherwise understand in less meaningful ways. Even the etymology of the words expressive and to express suggests the notion that meaning must be squeezed or expressed out of an experience. On this basis we learn to give art a second look, often discovering more by approaching the same work from different points of view. (p. 71)

Carpenter and Langston (2004) draw an analogy when they compare art educators and students to architects and contractors:

> Students will always need to know about and how to execute various art skills and techniques, just as an architect needs a wealth

of skills in order to draft plans for the contractor to follow. The architect must be aware of the diverse needs of the world in order to create meaningful dwellings that make relevant connections to the lives of the future homeowners. The architect conceives the structures, which in the art classroom is found in district curriculum guides and individual unit plans designed by teachers. Both contractors and art educators are tasked with breathing life into curriculum guides and unit plans. Contractors who believe that they are creating a home and not just a house are bonded with art educators who believe that they are not just teaching students how to draw. Instead, these art educators empower students to physically manifest thoughts, dreams, desires, and their voices in the world. (pp. 75-76)

In conclusion, your voice as a teacher matters. You have both a personal and professional life to negotiate for yourself and your students. You also help others gain access to their own knowledge about the curriculum of life. This is why Janesick (2004) encourages her students to construct a personal journal, "if for no other reason than to learn to write, reflect, and reinvent their ideas" (p. 57). Janesick suggests that journals are "one of the most democratic of art works, as it is easy for any of us to get a pen and paper. It is the singular act of writing a journal that enables thinking to advance, turn around, reflect upon itself, and question the existing order of things" (pp. 57-58).

## Issues of Quality Are a Pattern: Standards and Evidence

Planning for instruction is hard work. When you plan, you design multiple ways for your learners to access the content of the lesson. As you begin, you will be able to plan one way to educate for health. But eventually, you will be able to plan multiple ways to educate for health.

Planning focuses on a balance of concepts and skills, which is stated in the form of a question for the planner: What will students know and be able to do as a result of the lesson? The National Health Education Standards (NHES) shown in figure 5.6 are a framework for curriculum development in health education. The NHES outline eight standards for what students should know and be able to do at the end of preK-12 schooling. These standards will help you plan your lessons because they list developmental targets—known as performance indicators—for the health-related concepts and skills to be taught at different grade levels. The first two standards focus on health content knowledge, and the other six standards focus on skill development.

## National Health Education Standards: Achieving Excellence

The National Health Education Standards provide a framework for aligning curriculum, instruction, and assessment practices for preK-12 students. As a result of health education, students will be able to do the following:

1. Comprehend concepts related to health promotion and disease prevention to enhance health.

2. Analyze the influence of family, peers, culture, media, technology, and other factors on health behaviors.

3. Demonstrate the ability to access valid health information and products and services to enhance health.

4. Demonstrate the ability to use interpersonal communication skills to enhance health and avoid or reduce health risks.

5. Demonstrate the ability to use decision-making skills to enhance health.

6. Demonstrate the ability to use goal-setting skills to enhance health.

7. Demonstrate the ability to practice health-enhancing behaviors and avoid or reduce health risks.

8. Demonstrate the ability to advocate for personal, family, and community health.

**Figure 5.6**    The National Health Education Standards are a framework for curriculum development in health education.

Reprinted with permission from *National Health Education Standards: Achieving Excellence*, 2nd ed. © 2007 American Cancer Society, Inc., http://cancer.org/NHES. All rights reserved.

Brooks (2002) notes that we expect performance standards from chefs, journalists, attorneys, musicians, and accountants, to name a few. These professionals have creations, publications, performances, and practices that grow out of standards accepted by their disciplines, including certain certifications, licensures, or registries. In health education, our standards for curriculum design are developmentally planned for preK-12 learners. However, there are also professional standards for you to accomplish at the university, depending on your plans to work with children in preK-3 settings or with youth in grades four through nine. These professional standards, shown in table 5.3, are ways for you to think and act as a professional who will educate for health.

There are many ways to write a lesson plan. Several types of examples are shown in figures 5.7 through 5.10 as a guide. Once you plan and implement one of your lessons, you can try to convert your plans to

## Table 5.3   Professional Preparation Standards for PreK-3 and Grades 4-9

| Professional thinking and action skills for working with children preK-3 | Professional thinking and action skills for working with youth grades 4-9 |
|---|---|
| ❏ Communicate the concepts and purposes of health education.<br>❏ Assess the needs and interests of elementary students.<br>❏ Plan elementary school health instruction.<br>❏ Implement elementary school health instruction.<br>❏ Evaluate the effectiveness of elementary school health instruction. | ❏ Communicate the essential purposes of school health education.<br>❏ Collaborate with health education specialists in assessing the health behaviors of young adolescents.<br>❏ Participate in schoolwide, cross-curricular planning that focuses on the healthy development of young adolescents.<br>❏ Actively participate in the health education of young adolescents.<br>❏ Participate in evaluating the effectiveness of health education for young adolescents.<br>❏ Work collaboratively with all professionals in implementing a coordinated school health program.<br>❏ Serve as a resource person to young adolescents regarding their healthy development.<br>❏ Serve as an advocate for school health education and the well-being of young adolescents. |

Column 1 source: Joint Committee of the Association for the Advancement of Health Education and American School Health Association (1992).

Column 2 source: Joint Committee of the Association for the Advancement of Health Education, American School Health Association, National Middle School Association, American Association of School Administrators, and Council of Chief State School Officers (1996).

other formats so you have practice organizing your ideas for instruction. Keep in mind that the different structures of your lesson plans will have an effect on how your students learn. Figures 5.8 and 5.10 include the National Health Education Standards as a framework for your lesson design. To practice a health-enhancing behavior, your students will need a repertoire that includes declarative knowledge (e.g., benefits of sleep) *and* procedural knowledge (e.g., goal setting) in a particular context (e.g., when faced with homework or a favorite media program).

## Aesthetics Help Build Curriculum Thinking

Blumenfeld-Jones (2004) states the following about aesthetics:

> Dancers often think of themselves as clay to be molded by the choreographer. While the dancers produce the motions, it is the choreographer who directs what is kept, what is discarded, what modifications occur, and so forth. . . . By extension, what can be said for the choreographer can be equally said for the painter, playwright, theater director, sculptor, and conceptual artist. Each is a dictator within her/his domain. (p. 52)

Blumenfeld-Jones (2004) suggests a strong parallel between a good curriculum leader as someone who controls the curriculum team, similar to how a "choreographer controls dancers, a theater director controls actors and playwrights, or a painter controls paint and canvas" (p. 53). However, he prefers a curriculum leader who *facilitates* a democratic curriculum process and "uses aesthetic thinking to foster an aesthetic curriculum" (p. 55). He also suggests that "we must develop skill through careful study of the senses, that is to say, careful study of how to use the senses to make sense of experience and careful practice at using what we have come to know" (p. 54).

In summary, my basic assumption when writing this book is that healthy living includes both a personal and professional perspective. When we educate for health, we start with a microview on personal health patterns, then broaden the scope—even the vision—to include a macroview of ecological patterns of people (e.g., interpersonal and intrapersonal), places (e.g., institutions and community), and things (e.g., policy). To this end, you are encouraged to know the vision and mission statements of the school (or educational organization) where you work.

This chapter positions health education concerns as professional preparation issues and advocates for boundary-crossing work between education and health to support children and youth. There are natural pathways between the intrapersonal and interpersonal levels of the ecological model. How you interpret your role as a professional who educates for health can also be organized by the contextual model of human expertise. Plans, philosophy, pedagogy, and principles of practice are four of the many sources of knowledge you will come to know and make from your place in the world as you educate for health.

## Constructivist Pre-Lesson-Plan Template

Choose a lesson that you will soon teach in your own classroom. For that lesson, answer the following questions using the information from this book.

*Step 1:* **Planning for the learning using declarative and procedural objectives**

*What are your objectives for the lesson?*

Declarative objectives (what students will know)

1.

2.

3.

Procedural objectives (what students will be able to do)

1.

2.

3.

*Step 2:* **How will you use the human senses to introduce the learning?**

Visual:

Auditory:

Olfactory:

Touch:

Taste:

*Step 3:* **To which modalities are you teaching? How are you doing this?**

Visual:

Auditory:

Kinesthetic:

*Step 4:* **Information processing**

What will you do to ensure that students link new knowledge to old knowledge?

---

**Figure 5.7**  Lesson plan option 1 for health education.

### *Step 4:* Information Processing *(continued)*

Generate an internal representation of the new knowledge through graphic organizers.

---

### *Step 5:* Working memory

How will you ensure that students make better use of specific memory lanes?

Semantic memory:

Episodic memory:

Procedural memory:

### *Step 6:* Assessment

How will you communicate your learning expectations to your students?

---

**Figure 5.7**   *(continued)*

# Lesson Preplanning Outline

Topic of lesson: _____ Concept of lesson: _____ Grade level: ____

Personal or social skill of lesson:

__ decision making

__ goal setting

__ stress management

__ communication

__ conflict resolution

What National Health Education Standard(s) and Performance Indicators do you plan to address with this lesson?

_____

Generalization (take-home message):

_____

Turn the generalization into a guiding question for opening and closing the lesson:

_____

| Content | Evidence-based instructional strategies | Student assessments (e.g., in-class activities and assignments) |
|---------|------------------------------------------|----------------------------------------------------------------|
|         |                                          |                                                                |

**Figure 5.8** Lesson plan option 2 for health education.

## Lesson Implementation Plan

## Phases

### Activate Prior Knowledge

Call to mind what is known about a topic before proceeding with new information.

This phase also focuses on attention of the learner.

### Set the Context

Set the objectives and expectations for the lesson.

Use advanced organizers to provide an overview or "big picture" of the lesson and how it fits into a larger scheme.

### Instruction

Use demonstration, simulation, role-play, or direct teaching.

Engage learners in inquiry or other forms of active learning.

Use cooperative learning or individual learning.

### Check for Understanding

Conduct a formal assessment to ensure that learners have grasped the main points of the lesson.

### Practice and Apply

Use guided or independent practice.

Apply knowledge to products, performances, or processes.

Transfer learning and apply it to new and different situations.

### Closure

Bring lesson to formal conclusion.

Refocus on the lesson's objectives.

Foreshadow the next lesson.

---

**Figure 5.9** Lesson plan option 3 for health education.

# Lesson Implementation Schedule

Habit of health: _____ Habit of mind: _____ Grade level: _____

What National Health Education Standard(s) and Performance Indicators do you plan to address with this lesson?

_____

_____

| Lesson structure and time needed | Content of lesson | Student actions<br>*Do not write*<br>*"Students will . . ."* | Materials needed |
|---|---|---|---|
| *Introduction*<br><br>**Time** | • Greet students.<br>• Tell the lesson goal.<br>• Write the guiding question of the lesson on the board (and here): | | |
| *Entry point*<br><br>**Time** | | | |
| *Midpoint*<br><br>**Time** | | | |
| *Endpoint*<br><br>**Time** | | | |

**Figure 5.10**  Lesson plan option 4 for health education.

## CHAPTER FEATURES

### Principles of Practice

• Multiple health perspectives inform the ecological model: health sciences, health behavior, health education, and health communication. Each of these subdisciplinary perspectives can be thought of as an interpretation of the field.

• The interpersonal level of the ecological model in public health is linked by the interpersonal learning style in public education, which forms a cross-disciplinary bridge that connects health theory with education and educational theory with health.

• Learning styles have been explained as "four windows of opportunity" for accessing and interpreting information. As you gain in expertise as a professional who will educate for health, you need to be adaptable and flexible in accessing and communicating health-related information through all four learning styles. Educating for health through all four learning styles increases the opportunities for more people to learn about health.

• When designing, the structure and function of your planned educational lessons, curricula, and programs will help others seek an aesthetic quality of life. There are many functional and aesthetic ways to structure lessons in health education.

• You will weave your personal stories with professional theories to educate for health. Your personal and professional philosophies will be constructed from difference sources of knowledge. Sources of knowledge frame the outer level of the contextual model of human expertise, a modified version of the ecological model used in public health. Plans, philosophy, pedagogy, and principles of practice are four of the many sources of knowledge that highlight "what you know and what you do" in a particular context (e.g., institution or community) to make a difference in the world. Someday your own students will contribute to the world in similar ways.

### Teacher Voices

Following is a student teacher's reflection on her third week of teaching an eighth-grade health education class:

When I arrived at school on Friday morning, I was excited to start the day because the day before had gone so well. I had planned to do a quick demonstration of the chemicals in a cigarette and secondhand smoke, followed by a discovery learning activity. The demonstration was something that Mrs. Falk had done in the past, and something that I thought was going to be really fun for the students to see. Outside, I had attached a cigarette to the end of a dish soap bottle, which held some cotton balls. I lit the cigarette and squeezed the bottle to "smoke" the cigarette and, while that was going on, held a two-liter pop bottle over the burning end of the cigarette to catch the secondhand smoke. When we went back inside to discuss what we had just seen, the students were amazed at how much the cotton balls had turned to a yellowish brown color when they absorbed all the tar and were also amazed at the amount of secondhand smoke in the bottle. This part of the lesson went well as planned and proved to be effective for the students.

The discovery learning part of the lesson did not go as well as I had hoped it would. I had the class get with a partner, and then I handed out a few different printed resources along with a worksheet to fill out. Many of the students complained that they couldn't find the answers to the questions, and I had to keep reminding them that all the answers they needed could be found somewhere in the packet, and if they couldn't find them there, they could be found in the notes from earlier in the week, or in the book. After the third period, I was frustrated. The demonstration was going well, but the discovery learning activity was not. While discussing with Mrs. Falk during the plan period, I expressed that I was frustrated because the students simply were not putting any effort toward their work. To try to combat this, for the next period, I assigned the students a partner, instead of letting them pick their own, in hopes that they would stay on task a little more. Also, I handed out the information to them before handing out the worksheet, and told them to take some time and read through the information—so that they had an idea of what it was about—and told them that the worksheet would be a lot easier if they did this. This helped a little bit, but the last two periods always prove to be the most difficult to teach, especially on a Friday. I would be slightly hesitant to try something like this again. I think it is a great idea to have students find information out for themselves, but I think I would have to try to find another way to make it more interesting and keep the students on task.

*Abby Milbratz, Miami University Health Education Alumna, 2005*

## Seeds of Growth:
## Signs, Symbols, and Patterns of Living and Learning

1.   In your learning journal, reflect and write about Parker Palmer's quote: "In every story I have heard, good teachers share one trait: a strong sense of personal identity infuses their work" (1998, p. 10). In what way is that true of you? In what way is it not?

2.   In your learning journal, reflect and write about Nepo's (2005) quote: "All the spiritual traditions agree that the atom of the sacred is the moment. In this way, living with the sacred means opening ourselves to each moment. . . .

Our job as human beings, then, is to be born again each instant and to die again each instant. For it seems that life is an endless series of births, deaths, and small resurrections through which we are renewed" (pp. 67-68).

3.   In your learning journal, reflect and write about the reciprocal nature of teaching and learning in the context of Nepo's quote: "It's very much like the nature of water. We can't say, 'I'd prefer the hydrogen only, please.' Once you separate its elements, it is no longer water, no longer quenching. It is the same with joy and suffering. Together they form the water of life, and it is the gift of feeling keenly that allows us to drink from that source. Once we try to separate the joy from the sorrow, it is no longer life, no longer essential" (pp. 33-34).

## Web Links for Living and Learning

The National Health Education Standards (Joint Committee on NHES, 2007) were developed by a joint committee of education and health professionals from a wide variety of institutions. The American Association for Health Education (www.aahperd.org/AAHE); the American School Health Association (www.ashaweb.org); the American Public Health Association (www.apha.org); and the Society of State Directors of Health, Physical Education and Recreation (http://wg.thesociety.org) partnered on the writing project. Visit these different organizations online, as well as the American Cancer Society (www.cancer.org), which sponsored the project, to find background information on the curriculum-writing process and sample lessons using the National Health Education Standards for a particular age or grade level.

## Books for Living and Learning

*What I Like About Me! A Book Celebrating Differences* (Zobel-Nolan, 2005) is rich with kinesthetic flaps, colors, textures, rhythm, and rhyme. Analyze this picture book for its multiple language elements, also known as the signs, symbols, and patterns of multiple intelligences. How would you write a picture book about you? What language elements would you use to define your role as a professional who educates for health? Using the contextual model of human expertise, highlight what "sources of knowledge" you already know and what you are able to do to make a difference in the world.

# Ways to Design: Curriculum and Pedagogical Frameworks

6

For when a canoe drifts left or right, or gets stuck in the roots of an old willow, it is not wrong or evil or lacking in character. It is just being a canoe. Likewise, our rush to judge ourselves and others for what goes wrong, or not as we planned, is a distraction from engaging the nature of living, which is drifting and steering. With discernment but without judgment, the human journey is one of steering our way back to center over and over.

© by Mark Nepo, *The Exquisite Risk: Daring to Live an Authentic Life,* 2005

Teachers are interpreters of patterns. You will help young people seek patterns and rhythms in their personal health-related habits as you teach the curriculum or guide children to communicate effectively. As you gain experience through practice, you will become efficient in pattern making. The teacher's role as a guide on the side helps learners to be investigators who probe and discover patterns for self and other peers. For it is in the telling of their own discoveries that young people grow more knowledgeable. Using words, pictures, numbers, body language, rhythms, and environmental cues helps learners increase their communication repertoire by expressing what is known about a health topic, concept, or skill. When we educate for health, we use a variety of communication elements in order to give greater access to the health information. Although we may open or block the door to learning for certain young people, we must also teach them how to communicate for themselves as active participants in the exchange of information, not just passive recipients. This is why cooperative learning and peer education are valued as pedagogies—because the learners do the teaching. Both of these pedagogies of engagement lend themselves to inquiry-based approaches to learning.

The ability to observe and experience patterns in your own communication, both verbal and nonverbal, is a vital skill of any teacher. As you move into the disciplinary course work that enables you to become a teacher, search for ways to increase your content knowledge in that discipline, including the many ways in which that discipline can be communicated in a metalanguage of words, pictures, numbers, body language, rhythms, and environmental cues. In addition, look for similarities between two disciplines in both content knowledge (curriculum) and pedagogical knowledge (instruction), like I have done in bringing education and health together in this text. This helps you see cross-disciplinary patterns when educating for health.

Let's take a moment to see how conceptual patterns can emerge between health and other academic disciplines from a content (curriculum) perspective. In social studies, the historical questions of what, where, why, when, and with whom are excellent cues to action for studying the personal *story* of healthy behavior. In science, the focus on *change* in living organisms, including how plants, animals, and humans interact and adapt to their environments through a change process or metamorphosis, can captivate young people. In language arts, literacy approaches aimed at accessing and decoding texts in print and nonprint formats can help us identify health-related messages and themes. Using poetry, stories, film, and documentaries can help us motivate and inspire young people to do something about their health and well-being in the context of their *language* and culture. In math, the ability to see *patterns* in numerical data and in shapes enhances our learners' ability to practice habits of health in a systematic way.

Besides seeing patterns in content across disciplines, we can also look for patterns in how we teach across disciplines. This chapter will help you look for patterns in your pedagogy by using evidence-based instructional strategies. When Marzano, Pickering, and Pollock (2001) conducted a meta-analysis on 40 years of educational research, they identified nine instructional strategies that resulted in higher effects on student learning. These evidence-based instructional strategies are an effective way to give your students access to the health-related concepts and skills that you want them to know and be able to do. Your potential as an effective educator depends on your ability to learn and use your pedagogy in service to your students, not as the focal point to what you do. Darling-Hammond and Sykes (1999) also remind us that the quality of your instruction (i.e., your effectiveness in pedagogy) will determine how well your students will learn.

In a study by Wright, Horn, and Sanders (1997), the quality of a teacher determined how well students achieved in the classroom. In one year, effective teachers were associated with student achievement gains of 53 percentile points, but the least effective teachers were associated with student achievement gains of only 14 percentile points. When looking at the cumulative effects over 3 years between students taught by least-effective teachers versus students taught by most-effective teachers, the former were associated with student achievement gains of 29 percentile points but the latter were associated with student achievement gains of 84 percentile points. So certainly your effectiveness as a teacher makes a difference in the learning outcomes of your students! We now return to a discussion of constructivism and its relationship to pedagogy.

## Epistemology of Constructivism and Its Relationship to Pedagogy

Constructivism is, after all, an epistemology. Leamnson (1999) suggests the following:

> The desirable outcome of a well-reasoned philosophy is to produce an effective pedagogy, where pedagogy is not synonymous with method or technique. Pedagogy includes everything a teacher is and does when teaching and getting ready to teach. Methods and techniques are narrow and specific while one's pedagogy is more holistic. A technique might be found effective by one particular teacher, for a particular group of students, to teach a certain specific content. A good pedagogy selects what is appropriate and is not wedded to a method, no matter how innovative or popular. (p. 8)

According to Bredeson (2003), a view of pedagogy must take into account who is being taught: "An educator's expert knowledge cannot be reduced to a set of isolated skills and bits of technical knowledge. Instead, professional expertise is determined by how knowledge and skills are applied in situations of practice" (p. 35). He goes on to say that "a new mix of students and setting requires the teacher to use his knowledge and skills in ways that meet the demands of the new situation, not in simple replication of previous practice" (pp. 35-36).

## Pedagogical Content Knowledge

In 1986, Shulman developed a new framework for teacher education by introducing the concept of pedagogical content knowledge (PCK). Rather than dichotomize the education of teachers as being either content or pedagogy, Shulman suggests that these two types of knowledges be integrated to prepare teachers to teach more effectively. This encouraged educators to teach pedagogy and content together in courses instead of teaching pedagogy apart from subject matter. In fact, Shulman (1987) promotes PCK as "an understanding of how particular topics, problems, or issues are organized, presented, and adapted to the diverse interests and abilities of learners, and presented for instruction" (p. 8).

Shulman (1986, 1987) and Veal and MaKinster (1999) outline pedagogical content knowledge as a synthesis of three knowledge bases: subject matter knowledge, pedagogical knowledge, and contextual knowledge. Marzano et al. (1997) named these knowledge bases declarative knowledge (i.e., knowledge to know), procedural knowledge (i.e., knowledge to do), and contextual knowledge (i.e., knowledge to know and do in a context). Gagnon and Collay (2006) suggest using the following question prompts for constructivist lesson plans: What will your learners take out the door? How will your learners show what they know?

In chapter 4, I outlined declarative knowledge as the building blocks of facts, topics, concepts, generalizations, principles, models, and theories, and procedural knowledge as the building blocks of skills, strategies, techniques, methods, procedures, and processes. In chapter 5, I outlined the role of people, places, and things in my contextual model of human expertise. This model honors contextual knowledge by the way people interact with others in different institutions in certain places in the world. We educate for health when we make a difference in the world through our pedagogy, philosophy, presentations, performances, products, programs, principles, publications, props, and procedures. Hence, each of us can make a difference in the world when we share our expertise with others in a certain context.

In this text, types of declarative knowledge include *facts* about the human senses; the *topics* of exercise, nutrition, relationships, sleep, safety, and hygiene, known as habits of health; *concepts* of education, health, philosophy, and pedagogy; the wellness and ecological *models*; constructivist *principles;* and learning styles *theory,* multiple intelligences *theory,* and constructivist *theory.* Types of procedural knowledge include health-related *skills* called habits of mind; *processes* known as information processing; and pedagogical *processes* known as evidence-based instructional *strategies.* When you learn how to combine declarative and procedural knowledge together into pedagogical content knowledge, you will be modeling your competence (and expertise) in contextual knowledge.

You may ask how you begin such a sophisticated task of instructional design. You begin by learning terminology and examples for each type of knowledge, while interacting with your students and other colleagues as you implement your designs. The more you talk about, rethink, and redesign your instructional plans while teaching different students, the better you will become at constructing meaning about what your students should know and be able to do in certain institutions and places in their changing world.

Marzano and colleagues (1997) show that procedural knowledge takes more time to learn than declarative knowledge, but that each is informed by the other. Since in this chapter we focus on a type of procedural knowledge—called evidence-based instructional strategies (EBIS)— keep in mind that you will need lots of practice in this form of pedagogy. Specifically, you will need to take the time to practice implementing the nine different strategies in table 6.1. This, of course, requires that you first learn what each of the strategies is and then begin to use them as an action of your work.

## Evidence-Based Instructional Strategies in Health Education

You will especially need time and experience in combining EBIS (your pedagogy) with what your students should know and be able to do, e.g., habits of health and habits of mind. As you gain expertise in educating for health, you will be able to help young people practice their cognitive skills—habits of mind, e.g., decision making, goal setting, communication, stress management, and conflict resolution—while you use pedagogical strategies—EBIS, e.g., identifying similarities and differences, summarizing and note taking, reinforcing effort and providing recognition, homework and practice, nonlinguistic representations, cooperative learning, setting objectives and providing feedback, generating and testing hypotheses, and questions, cues, and advanced organizers. Whew! You will also focus on different habits of health, e.g., exercise, nutrition, relationships, sleep, safety, and hygiene, to generate student

Table 6.1   **Categories of Evidence-Based Instructional Strategies (EBIS) That Affect Student Achievement**

| Category | Average effect size | Percentile gain | Number of effect sizes | Standard deviation |
|---|---|---|---|---|
| Identifying similarities and differences | 1.61 | 45 | 31 | 0.31 |
| Summarizing and note taking | 1.00 | 34 | 179 | 0.50 |
| Reinforcing effort and providing recognition | 0.80 | 29 | 21 | 0.35 |
| Homework and practice | 0.77 | 28 | 134 | 0.36 |
| Nonlinguistic representations | 0.75 | 27 | 246 | 0.40 |
| Cooperative learning | 0.73 | 27 | 122 | 0.40 |
| Setting objectives and providing feedback | 0.61 | 23 | 408 | 0.28 |
| Generating and testing hypotheses | 0.61 | 23 | 63 | 0.79 |
| Questions, cues, and advance organizers | 0.59 | 22 | 1,251 | 0.26 |

From R.J. Marzano, D.J. Pickering, and J.E. Pollock, 2001, *Classroom instruction that works: Research-based strategies for increasing student achievement* (Alexandria, VA: Association for Supervision and Curriculum Development), 7. Reprinted by permission of McREL. All rights reserved.

interest in learning. Since these different habits of health are actually behaviors, you can call your class ACTions for health!

Now would you agree that you will need patience and practice with lots of trial and error to educate for health? Of course! That is what makes teaching so interesting and dynamic. Just when you have found an effective way to help kids practice managing their stress through exercise or adequate sleep, you are surprised to learn that you have a student who uses English as a second language or you have a student who is gifted and needs a curriculum extension or adaptation. Regarding your growing sophistication with instructional design, Leamnson (1999) suggests that "if the desired synapses are to be stabilized, and so made available for future use, they need to be used repeatedly, in different contexts, and with intervals between" (p. 73).

In this next section, I will give you some examples of how to integrate EBIS, habits of mind, and habits of health. I will italicize the pedagogy that follows to help you focus on how to implement EBIS, which is your skill set to practice when educating for health. Please note that EBIS serves as a metacognitive overlay to your entire instructional design. That is, you don't start planning your instruction based on an EBIS. Instead, you start planning instruction with what your students should know and be able to do as healthy human beings. How you get there, i.e., your evidence-based instructional strategies, becomes the interlocking fingers for integrating the habits of health with the habits of mind.

For example, if you want seventh grade students to be able to make effective decisions when choosing what to eat for breakfast, you might have them use a *compare and contrast strategy* for which cereal will give them the least amount of simple sugars and which milk will give them the least amount of fat. For third grade students, you can send home a checklist of foods that contain calcium and ask kids and their parents or caregivers to help them choose one serving of calcium-rich foods for each of their meals on a Saturday or Sunday for homework. When they return to the classroom on Monday, you can have them write a three-sentence *summary* of what they ate for breakfast, lunch, and dinner. You can then have them *take notes* while you explain the importance of calcium for bone, teeth, and heart health. Complete the lesson by having students exchange papers for a *cooperative learning* activity in which each student reads and *gives feedback* on whether there were three different facts written down about calcium on their classmate's paper. You can give *homework and additional practice* on calcium by asking students to bring in an empty food container or package with calcium listed on the food label. By requiring students to eat the food containing calcium before they bring an empty container or package to class, you are *reinforcing effort and achievement* for healthy nutrition. Hence, a habit of health, e.g., nutrition, is practiced along with a habit of mind, e.g., decision making.

Let's take one more example of using EBIS as the interlocking fingers between a habit of health and a habit of mind. In fifth grade, you can help students select facts on how to make new multicultural friends from a valid and reliable health brochure, textbook, or Web site. Help students organize the factual information into a *graphic organizer* (also known as a nonlinguistic representation) with a theme on friendships (or relationships). So students will *practice* their communication skills in a *cooperative learning* activity, place the graphic organizers on a bulletin board or on the wall down a hallway where they can do a gallery walk to show their work. One-half of the students can get *recognition* by standing next to their graphic organizers on the wall and interacting with classmates who stop by and practice *asking questions or using cues* for good listening. This assignment integrates a habit of health, e.g., relationships, with a habit of mind, e.g., communication, when students interact with their classmates and their teacher. You can culminate the activity by asking students *to generate and test a hypothesis,* i.e., a general rule, on how communication between their classmates might change when they are on the playground or on the school bus going home, including *summarizing* how to make a new multicultural friend.

## Evidence-Based Instructional Strategies Are Tools and Patterns for All Disciplines

When educating for health, patterns emerge around evidence-based instructional strategies. Educators of all disciplines should be able to model these strategies and explain their processes effectively so that their learners will be able to recognize these metacognitive strategies themselves as they gain in cognitive development and sophistication. Each of the evidence-based instructional strategies is briefly explained in the list that follows and more fully described in Marzano et al. (1997). You can also view many summative examples of these strategies in appendix 6.1 at the end of this chapter.

1. Identifying similarities and differences involves
   - comparing,
   - classifying,
   - creating metaphors, and
   - creating analogies.

2. Summarizing and note taking can be done using different frameworks, which include
   - the narrative frame,
   - the topic-restriction-illustration frame,
   - the definition frame,
   - the argumentation frame,
   - the problem-solution frame, and
   - the conversation frame.

3. Reinforcing effort and providing recognition are best done through
   - showing the connection between effort and achievement and
   - using symbolic recognition rather than tangible rewards.

4. Homework and practice are guided by the following principles:
   - Amount varies by grade level.
   - Parent involvement should be minimal.
   - Teacher should give feedback on all assigned homework.
5. Nonlinguistic representations include many types of graphic organizers, such as figures, tables, and charts.

   Nonlinguistic representations also include many types of thinking or mind maps (Hyerle, 2004).
6. Cooperative learning can include student interactions in
   - informal groups,
   - formal groups, and
   - base groups.
7. Setting objectives and providing feedback involve
   - adapting instructional objectives so they reflect student learning objectives and
   - using specific goals rather than general goals.
8. Generating and testing hypotheses involve
   - the application of knowledge,
   - using deductive approaches in which a principle is provided and then students generate and test a hypothesis based on the principle, and
   - using inductive approaches in which students discover a principle and then generate hypotheses or use a general rule to make a prediction.
9. Questions, cues, and advance organizers help students use what they already know about a topic to improve their learning. This involves
   - using prior knowledge in addition to new information to learn something new,
   - asking thoughtful questions about people, things, actions, events, and other ideas, and
   - preparing students for what they will learn in the near future.

In his book *Knowledge as Design*, David Perkins (1986) uses four guiding questions to investigate the nature of any design: What is its purpose (or purposes)? What is its structure (and parts)? What are model cases

## Evidence-Based Instructional Strategy: Nonlinguistic Representations

***What types of nonlinguistic representation structures are there?***

There are two main types of nonlinguistic representations:

- Graphic organizers (Marzano et al., 1997)
- Thinking maps (Hyerle, 2004)

***You should use a nonlinguistic representation***

- to show relationships between ideas,
- with learners at the fourth grade and above, and
- with coaching or explicit practice to learn each type of structure.

***What is the purpose of the nonlinguistic representation strategy?***

Graphic organizers and mind maps have multiple purposes:

- They put ideas into visual form (pictures and graphics).
- They show your thinking process.
- They develop your ideas.
- They organize your thinking patterns into a structure that enhances memory.

***What are model cases or examples of the nonlinguistic representation strategy?***

There are many examples of nonlinguistic representations. Graphic organizers (Marzano et al., 1997) include the following:

- Descriptive pattern organizer
- Time sequence pattern organizer
- Cause and effect pattern organizer
- Episode pattern organizer
- Generalization or principle pattern organizer
- Concept pattern organizer

Thinking maps (Hyerle, 2004) include the following:

- Tree map to classify and group
- Circle map to define and put in context
- Bubble map to describe and list adjectives

---

**Figure 6.1** Design questions for evidence-based instructional strategies.

- Double bubble map to compare and contrast
- Multiflow map for cause and effect
- Flow map for sequential order
- Brace map for whole objects and parts
- Bridge map for seeing analogies

### What is the evidence that the nonlinguistic representation strategy is useful?

Nonlinguistic representation strategies help you do the following:

- Link information and ideas together.
- Reduce and organize information, using graphic organizers.
- Generate new ideas and see your thinking grow, using thinking maps.
- Show unique patterns in your thinking.

---

**Figure 6.1**    *(continued)*

---

or examples of it? What is the evidence that explains and evaluates it? For the purposes of this chapter, I have made the following modifications to Perkins' questions to use in studying the nine evidence-based instructional strategies:

- What types of _____ structures are there?
- What is the purpose of the _____ strategy?
- What are model cases or examples of the _____ strategy?
- What is the evidence that the _____ strategy is useful?

For an in-depth look at how Perkins' four design questions can be used to organize one of these strategies (e.g., nonlinguistic representations), review figure 6.1. I would encourage you to apply Perkins' four design questions to each of the EBIS as a way to construct deeper meaning from these pedagogical tools. Feel free to draw upon the available academic literature to study each strategy, keeping developmental appropriateness for different age groups in mind.

# Theoretical Mapping of Three Learning Zones in Educating for Health

After reading an article by Spady (1994), I reflected on three major zones of learning, each more sophisticated than the last. In the traditional zone, typical subject matter content is considered. In the transitional zone, disciplines, contexts, and settings are transcended so that they are integrated and synthesized to make an interdisciplinary approach. An example of this might be health education, because it is an interdisciplinary field that draws on the fields of public health and public education. In the transformational zone, Spady suggests applications of growing complexity in real-life performance contexts.

In this text, I believe that learning styles theory, constructivist theory, and multiple intelligences theory are applications that cut across all disciplines, although they are not adequately addressed in all disciplines. This text shows how these three educational theories can be used in health education. In addition, this text highlights evidence-based instructional strategies as a new form of pedagogy to be used in health education. The fact that EBIS are another application of growing complexity in real-life performance contexts puts this text in a potential transformational zone, which is solely dependent on how other scholars in health education evaluate its merit and whether they begin to use these three theories and nine evidence-based instructional strategies as forms of declarative and procedural knowledge, respectively.

Currently, there are many excellent curriculum models in health education for children and youth. Curriculum models that are aligned with the National Health Education Standards (Joint Committee on NHES, 2007) are continually updating and changing, so curricula are beyond the scope of this book. However, this chapter has highlighted the advantages of using nine EBIS for improving student achievement. To date, no one has analyzed the use of evidence-based instructional strategies within evidence-based health education curricula from an instructional design perspective. I propose that the integration of these two approaches will be a promising way to increase the effectiveness of health education in preK-8 in the years to come. I invite you to take an interest in moving the profession forward with this in mind, so that we can educate for health with more effective and efficient approaches.

The next chapter will remind you that when you educate for health, you must ultimately use a relational pedagogy that focuses on your students and their command of health-related topics, concepts, and skills.

## CHAPTER FEATURES

### Principles of Practice

• When educating for health, professionals can organize their work by curriculum, instruction, and assessment. Other professionals organize content and pedagogy together and call it pedagogical content knowledge. Yet other professionals differentiate knowledge as declarative, procedural, and contextual.

• Knowledge as design forms the basis of how knowledge is organized and structured, how it functions, and whether it enhances learning and health for individuals or groups of learners.

• Evidence-based instructional strategies (EBIS) are the pedagogical tools used by professionals for improving student achievement across all content areas and across all grade levels. EBIS are a form of procedural knowledge because they are strategies. Procedural knowledge includes skills, strategies, methods, procedures, and processes.

• Evidence-based instructional strategies are another way to connect health education to the larger story of education. Professionals from all disciplines can use EBIS as an effective way to educate. EBIS serves as a metacognitive tool that helps to integrate the habits of health with the habits of mind when educating for health.

### Teacher Voices

What follows is an e-mail exchange between a novice and an expert teacher regarding different health education classes in a middle school.

*Novice:* I have come to the realization that some classes just don't participate very well. In the morning we do all kinds of discussion activities, and there is excellent participation, but in the afternoon it's like pulling teeth to get them to answer questions, or they all talk at once and nothing gets accomplished. So I'm learning that lesson adaptations just have to be made from class to class.

*Expert:* That's right, a key to effective teaching is one's ability to adapt and adjust to the learners. That may be the number one educational principle that helps us become good teachers. Nothing is ever the same (which is a very daunting generalization).

*Novice:* My morning classes have more discussion and group work, while my afternoon classes do things more individually. Also my morning classes take their time and do the assignments correctly. The afternoon classes rush through the assignments, so I have to have something extra planned for them; otherwise it turns into complete chaos.

   *Expert:* How much of this is due to energy levels from lunch or lack of sleep the night before? Did you ever think you would use different evidence-based instructional strategies in different classes within one day?

*Jennifer Lane, Miami University health education alumna, 2005,*
*with Valerie A. Ubbes, mentor and academic adviser*

## Seeds of Growth:
## Signs, Symbols, and Patterns of Living and Learning

   1.  As a professional who educates for health, you will be in constant planning mode. In your learning journal, reflect and write about how Nepo's (2005) quote helps you negotiate your work, rest, and play.

   We are taught at an early age to pull things apart in order to solve them, to break problems down to understand their parts. Yet in the terrain of spirit and relationship, in the sweet territory of compassion, we often need to let things in rather than break things down. So, the question each day becomes: When pressed by life, do I bridge or isolate? Do I reconnect the web of life and listen to its wisdom? Or do I make an island of every confusion as I try to solve its pain? (p. 22)

   2.  Reflect on a lesson you were recently taught in a university course. Which evidence-based instructional strategies were used? Write a brief narrative on how you were a passive participant or an active learner during the class session. Cite specific examples as evidence for your learning.

   3.  Either alone or in a cooperative learning group, create a template like the one found in figure 6.1 for the other evidence-based instructional strategies. Your professional expertise will not be based on your ability to incorporate these strategies in your lesson plans to use yourself. Eventually, your use of these strategies as tools for your students to learn about health will be the hallmark of the co-curriculum. You need to know how to use and model these strategies so your students can learn from you how to use them. Now, that is educating for health! If you teach using an evidence-based instructional strategy, you are doing the active learning, and your students are probably being passive learners. Keep planning for ways for your students to use EBIS so they can be active learners.

## Web Links for Living and Learning

Robert Marzano has posted several resources to help professionals understand his research on evidence-based instructional strategies. Go to www.middleweb.com/MWLresources/marzchat1.html to learn more about his research on EBIS, then find some Web sites of your own to get ideas for using

EBIS in planning your instructional lessons and units. For example, Haynes (2007) notes that English language learners (ELLs) become better writers if they begin with nonfiction writing that focuses on content information and vocabulary in a discipline. Since it takes ELLs longer to master academic language than it does to become fluent in social language, it is not a good idea to ask ELLs to write personal narratives or journal entries. Instead, structure classwork with graphic organizers so ELLs can use chunks of language to develop their writing skills. Haynes (2007) states, "Many students think about what they are going to write in their native language, then translate their thoughts into English. Some may even write in their native language first. This translated language, full of inaccurate verb tenses and incorrect sentence structures, often results in an unintelligible product" (p. 34). So use an EBIS to help make your lesson culturally (and linguistically) sensitive for these students.

## Books for Living and Learning

The book *Tools* (Morris & Heyman, 1998) takes us on a universal trip around the world to see how people use tools to make their lives easier. After reading the book, think about the tools you will use to educate for health. Either alone or in a cooperative learning group with your colleagues, create a picture book that shows the tools (electronic and nonelectronic) that are used in education and health. Reflect on the role of lesson plans as a pedagogical tool. How many pedagogical tools are concrete objects? Are there any pedagogical tools that generate abstract thoughts?

# Appendix 6.1 Evidence-Based Instructional Strategies (EBIS) Examples

- **Compare and Contrast Through Analogy and Metaphor**

## LEARNING STYLES

Silver, Strong, and Perini (2000) outline a model of four learning styles derived from the theories of Carl Jung and Isabel Briggs Myers.

### Mastery Learners

These learners prefer opportunities to observe, describe, memorize, and practice new learning to reach mastery. They appreciate teachers who present information and arrange for practice. They enjoy developing mastery of basic skills.

The metaphor for this learning style is a *clipboard*. The following elements would be valued by this learning style:

- Organization
- Structure
- Visual directions
- Clear closure
- Sequential learning
- Clear procedures
- Consistent routines
- Clear expectations

### Interpersonal

These learners prefer opportunities to socialize, describe feelings, empathize, and provide support and approval. They appreciate teachers who relate the content to them personally so they can recognize relevance and add meaning to their work.

The metaphor for this learning style is a *puppy*. The following elements would be valued by this learning style:

- Comfortable environment
- Encouraging atmosphere
- Supportive grouping

- Safe climate
- Respectful colleagues
- Empathetic listeners
- Sensitive peers

## Understanding

These learners prefer opportunities to summarize, classify, compare, contrast, and look for cause and effect. They appreciate teachers who provide information and then probe for explanations and reasons behind the facts. They think logically and analytically, seeking evidence to support their learning.

The metaphor for this learning style is a *microscope*. The following elements would be valued by this learning style:

- Discovery learning
- Analyzing concepts
- Deep exploration
- Discussions
- Focus on details
- Ownership

## Self-Expressive

These learners prefer opportunities for original, flexible, and elaborate thinking. They appreciate teachers who give them choices and facilitate their learning. They are innovative, creative learners.

The metaphor for this learning style is a *beach ball*. The following elements would be valued by this learning style:

- Variety of resources
- Adaptive environment
- Various manipulatives
- Spontaneity
- Extensions to activities
- Personal freedom

- Compare and Contrast Through Analogy and Metaphor
- Questions, Cues, and Advance Organizers

## PreK-8 DEVELOPMENTAL QUESTION 1

### How can you practice habits of health every day?

*Habits of health (ACTions)*

- Eating and drinking
- Exercising and playing
- Protecting (safety) and preventing (hygiene)
- Relating and interacting
- Sleeping, resting, and reflecting

## PreK-8 DEVELOPMENTAL QUESTION 2

### How can you use habits of mind to practice habits of health every day?

*Personal skills*

- Decision making: time to decide—productive? destructive?
- Goal setting: time planned for the future
- Stress management: taking care of problems

*Social skills*

- Communication: talking, listening, expressing
- Conflict resolution: getting along

*Note: Habits of mind are also called personal and social skills.

- Cooperative Learning
- Questions, Cues, and Advance Organizers

## APPOINTMENT WITH A COLLEAGUE

Please make an appointment with 12 different people in class—one for each hour on the clock. Be sure to record each other's name for an appointment time on your individual clocks. Make the appointment only if you both have an open slot at that hour on your clocks.

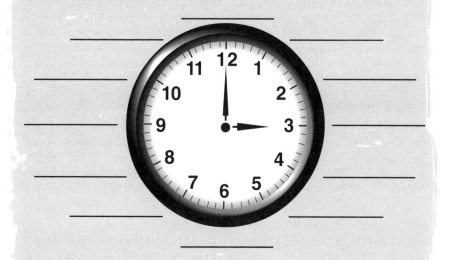

Please tape this paper inside a notebook so it is in class with you each day—if requested. Thank you!

Reprinted from Research for Better Teaching, Inc. (Bellows Hill Road, Carlisle, MA).

*(continued)*

*(continued)*

## DIRECTIONS AND QUESTION PROMPTS
## FOR THE COOPERATIVE LEARNING ACTIVITY

### Directions for Think, Pair, Share

• During a "think" cue, your instructor will prompt you to read one of the sample question prompts below. Write down very brief notes or points you plan to discuss with a colleague. Writing is an extended form of thinking.

• When given a "pair" cue, find a colleague at the designated appointment time and "share" your response to the designated question. Each person should talk and be heard for 5 minutes, then your roles are reversed. The goal is to engage *in dialogue,* not discussion, during your 10-minute appointment (total time). Please try to use a library voice so a pleasant environment for talking and listening is maintained.

### Sample Question Prompts

• When was the last time you wrote a song or poem to express your feelings and thoughts? Why is writing in these genres a good way to reveal your self-identity and growth potential? If you have not had this experience, discuss why youth should be given the space and time to do this (or not).

• What is one of the best books you have read? In what ways did the book communicate something "near and dear" to your heart or affirm a philosophical belief you hold? If you do not have a book to share, discuss why youth should be encouraged to choose their reading material in addition to required reading.

• What is the most recent question you asked to get more information, to understand something deeper, or to get to know someone better? Discuss the role of inquiry in maximizing your potential as a human being. How do we invite youth to engage in inquiry?

• What movie or television show gives you insight into who you are? Describe the scene or synopsis of the show briefly to reveal why you can identify with it so much. Would this movie or television show be appropriate for youth? Why or why not?

- Questions, Cues, and Advance Organizers
- Summarizing

**REFLECTION ON YOUR PERSONAL AND PROFESSIONAL LIFE**

*Think about and write a brief response for each question.*

What three words would you use to describe yourself as a student?

What three words would you use to describe yourself as a teacher?

What do you consider your greatest personal accomplishment?

What do you consider your greatest professional accomplishment?

What was the defining moment of your personal life?

What was the defining moment of your professional life?

What was the greatest challenge you faced in your personal life?

What was the greatest challenge you faced in your professional life?

What is your favorite activity outside of work?

What is your greatest indulgence?

What was the last book you read?

What was the last movie you liked?

What is your favorite work of art?

What is your favorite form of exercise?

If you could go anywhere on vacation, where would you go?

Where would you like to take your students to learn?

What is the best thing about being a teacher?

What is the hardest thing about being a teacher?

What would you most like to be remembered for?

How will your students remember you?

Adapted by permission of FORBES.com. © March 30, 2005 Forbes.com.

## COMPARISONS BETWEEN DIALOGUE, DISCUSSION, AND DEBATE

| *Dialogue*<br>The purpose of dialogue is to reach understanding. | *Discussion*<br>The purpose of discussion is to make a decision. | *Debate*<br>The purpose of debate is to argue successfully for my position over that of an opponent. |
|---|---|---|
| • I listen in order to understand.<br>• I listen for strengths so as to affirm and to learn from others.<br>• I speak for myself from my own understanding and experience.<br>• I ask questions to increase my understanding and the understanding of others.<br>• I allow others to complete their communications.<br>• I focus on others' words and feelings.<br>• I accept others' experiences as real and valid for them.<br>• I allow the expression of real feelings in myself and in others.<br>• I honor silence. | • I listen in order to understand options.<br>• I listen in order to compare strengths and weaknesses.<br>• I speak based on information and opinions about options.<br>• I ask questions to gather information on pros and cons of the options.<br>• I change the subject if I think I have enough information.<br>• I question others' facts, information, and opinions.<br>• I avoid expressing feelings.<br>• I consider silence a waste of time. | • I listen in order to argue against what I hear.<br>• I listen for weaknesses so as to discount and devalue.<br>• I speak based on my assumptions about others' positions or motives.<br>• I ask questions to trip up or to confuse.<br>• I interrupt or change the subject.<br>• I focus on the point I next want to make.<br>• I critique others' experiences as distorted or invalid.<br>• I express my feelings to manipulate others and deny that their feelings are legitimate.<br>• I use silence to gain advantage. |

Reprinted, by permission, from M. Treichel, 2006, *Evidence-based instructional strategies: Dialogue, discussion, and debate* (Columbus, OH: Ohio Peace Center).

- Setting Objectives and Providing Feedback
- Nonlinguistic Representations
- Summarizing

## SAMPLE RUBRICS FOR ASSESSING HEALTH-RELATED SKILLS

Use a rubric to see if a lesson objective is being done in sequential order or with all the subskills being practiced by the student. You can use this rubric at three levels:

- Self-assessment (student does a personal assessment)
- Peer assessment (student does a review of a peer)
- Expert assessment (teacher does the assessment of the student)

**Sample Rubric 1: "When Someone Bothers You" Skill**

Student's name _____ Date _____

Name of peer _____ Rechecked date _____

| Subskills | Exemplary | Accomplished | Developing | Beginning |
|-----------|-----------|--------------|------------|-----------|
| Tell the person what he or she did. | X | | | |
| What bothered you about what he or she did? | | X | | |
| What did you want him or her to do instead? | | X | | |

*(continued)*

*(continued)*

## Sample Rubric 2: "Listening" Skill

Use a checklist to see how many students can demonstrate the following subskills for listening. A simple check mark can indicate that a student modeled the subskill, or you can use + and – to show positive and negative effects of the skill. Use this rubric in multiple settings or contexts to see if students are nearing mastery of the skill.

| Student's name | Stop what you are doing. | Look at the person who is speaking. | Be quiet while the person is speaking. | Ask questions or comment on what is being said. |
|---|---|---|---|---|
| Carrie | + | + | + | + |
| Steve | – | – | + | + |
| Pat | – | + | + | – |

Context or setting:

____ classroom

____ cafeteria

____ recess

____ hallway

Rubric by V.A. Ubbes, 2002, *Subskill content from the Michigan Model for Health.* Available: http://www.emc.cmich.edu/mm/default.htm

- Compare and Contrast
- Nonlinguistic Representation
- Questions, Cues, and Advance Organizers

## QUESTION PROBES FOR REVIEWING A STORY

| Objective inquiry | Subjective inquiry |
| --- | --- |
| Who is the intended *audience* for the story? | With whom might you share the story? |
| What is the main *message* of the story? | What is your *interpretation* (point of view) of the main message of the story? |
| What is the *context* for the story? | In what *context* does the story apply to your life? |
| What is the *subtext* of the story? | What is at least one hidden *assumption* that you can "uncover" and explore beneath the surface so the story is more meaningful for you? |

Question probes might work best by asking an objective question from the first column, followed by a subjective question from the second column. This allows each row of questions to stimulate both a public discourse and personal meaning making.

# 7

# Ways to Build Relationships Between People and Their Ideas

For it makes a difference if we view the waters of the earth as seven separate oceans or one magnificent sea. It makes a difference if we view the lands of the earth as separate nations or one massive home. It makes a difference if we view those living on earth as separate peoples or one family or humankind. A liberating difference if we delineate between humans and animals and plants and stones or if we affirm the common thread of life in all things.

© by Mark Nepo, *The Exquisite Risk: Daring to Live an Authentic Life*, 2005

The major theme of this book is that philosophical and pedagogical patterns weave to form many different path*ways* leading to education and health. As I mentioned at the onset of our journey, I have purposely invested in the concepts and theories that are common to all disciplines, but I have shown you how to implement them in the context of health education. Metaphor after metaphor, analogy after analogy, and example after example, I have tried to guide you to the language of possibility using the elements of design (e.g., structure, function, and aesthetics). By using a personal narrative style, supported by expository expertise from learned scholars, I have tried to guide you in the rationale and vision to educate for health.

Our story of design began with a personal connection to the elements of structure, function, and aesthetics—the building blocks of design. When we want to tell the story of instructional or pedagogical design, we focus on concepts, topics, and skills within one or more professional disciplines. When we design interdisciplinary connections between health and other disciplines, we seek a common language around concepts. This allows professionals who educate for health to cross disciplinary boundaries to study, exchange, and weave their ideas through shared relationships.

You might be interested in patterns in mathematics, which can lead you to understand health-related patterns of human behavior known as habits of health. Mathematical patterns emerge through epidemiology, which give us the subdisciplinary study of health behavior. Although epidemiologists in public health often focus on high risk health behaviors of populations and their relationship to mortality, morbidity, and longevity, we have focused on the health-promoting behaviors known as habits of health. We can help young people realize frequency patterns of hours slept each night of the week, including bedtimes and wake-up times, by helping them identify their behavioral patterns (habits) through the concept of their daily story.

Story emerges from the subdisciplinary study of health communication. Historically, people shared information through verbal storytelling and eventually through written forms of information via flyers, leaflets, and newspapers. Newspaper journalists, and now broadcast journalists, continue to use the historical patterns of "who, what, where, when, why, and with whom" to tell human stories of social and historical significance. We can help young people tell stories and read about their personal health through these inquiry prompts too: *What* do you do *when* you see something on the Internet or on television that makes you feel uncomfortable? *Who* do you talk to about your feelings? *Where* do you go if you need help to solve a problem? *Why* do you tell someone? Many of these questions can inform our personal health decisions for any habit of health. The concept of story, from its etymological root *history* (and symbolically, *her*story), weaves the journey of humans into a curriculum of health and life.

When educating for health, you might also be drawn to the concept of language that helps humans communicate and be literate in different genres. Language advances the subdisciplinary study of health education that traditionally emerges in preK-12 school settings but also crosses over into many nonschool settings across the life span. We draw upon words, pictures, numbers, body language, rhythms, and environmental cues when we promote health with a developmental perspective. When we combine these language elements into unique health-promoting messages for people as they age, we can educate for health (not disease), as long as the recipients of those messages have the intention to act on those educational experiences. Sometimes, humans choose to act in harmful ways to form habitual patterns, but health education invites an exploration of our habits of *health* and habits of mind.

Health educators need to use a broad repertoire of different language elements to design lessons and curricula that are structured around learning styles, multiple intelligences, and health education theories that focus on sensory-motor, cognitive-behavioral principles of learning. When we educate young people through their formative years, it is critically important for us to model the cognitive skills (e.g., habits of mind) and healthful behaviors (e.g., habits of health) as grown-ups. We don't have to be perfect role models, but our own journey to health and well-being requires a philosophical awareness of our pedagogies of professional practice. To encourage learners to take messages about health seriously, we must also be instructional designers who bring art, music, and physical education approaches into health education so that kids want to come back again and again to engage their senses in learning about their personal health. By integrating a variety of language elements, curriculum concepts and skills, and evidence-based instructional strategies, we increase the "opportunity for unity" between people and our pedagogy.

Finally, we must take seriously the need to connect children and youth with their changing bodies and brains in health-enhancing, culturally sensitive, and developmentally appropriate ways. Remember that we began this book with the concept of metamorphosis, or change. Our human health is changed by personal and cultural influences, informed by environments which are health enhancing or harmful and risky. Change is observed as energy in the subdisciplinary study of health science. Patterns of cause and effect, growth and development, and balance and adaptations describe change of human beings within the ecosystems of the world. When we educate for health, we need not study disease of the human body so as to scare young people from their own shelter of structure and function before they have a disease. But we can invite an awe and appreciation for the human body and mind as a pathway to the experience of self-identity and self-care. By acknowledging the role of our human senses in information processing and learning, we enter the human body with respect and sensitivity, and when learners are ready, we move beyond the naming of body parts into an exploration of body systems and functions, which leads to an aesthetic appreciation of our human potential. In the meantime, we study the human body and mind by looking at the affects of foods, medicines, drugs, sunlight, and other objects on and in the human body. When we educate for health, we must be sensitive to the ways in which we "dis" the body around young people by telling stories and using language of disease, disorders, disabilities, and discomforts. There are more-than-adequate healthy pleasures that contribute to our quality of life. By building a respectful relationship to our bodies and brains through subjective, not merely objective, approaches to health science, we can create a whole generation of young people who love the structure and functions of their human form. By building a relationship with ourselves in the context of who we are, with the supportive role of what we do (through our habits of health and habits of mind), we may be able to understand the quantity and quality of changes we experience across the life span. Perhaps by exploring the role of nature and the environment, including our interactions with natural environments, we will find true comfort and pleasure on our journeys.

Ultimately, it is the ways in which we build relationships with people and their ideas that we form the disciplinary stories of education and health, including the subdisciplinary stories and connections between health behavior, health communication, health education, and health science. The rest of this chapter will explore the role of relationship as a macroconcept that connects us all.

As you explore the integration of your personal and professional stories throughout your life, remember to consciously focus on wellness as an adult who can negotiate multiple dimensions of health. If you focus on your intellectual health at the expense of your physical health, or if you favor your social health over your spiritual health, one or two of your health dimensions will grow out of balance. Greenberg (1985) suggests that your lopsided wellness wheel will continue to bump you along through life until you choose symmetry and wholeness in your daily living. Remember that it is the relationship between these five dimensions of health that forms your well-being. You must consciously cue yourself to integrate these different dimensions of health into your daily experiences and not to isolate only a few dimensions from the whole.

Honoring the multiple dimensions of health throughout your day at school, in the community, and at home will uncover your daily wellness or illness patterns. You will probably recognize the *dis*-ease of life if you continually ignore the concepts of moderation and balance. Often the warning signs and cues come from our five senses and five dimensions of health, but sometimes the pain comes from within the body before we have taken the time to notice and attend to our core knowledge. Wellness can't always prevent disease, disorders, and disabilities, but seeing health as well-being helps us to connect with the self in personal and private ways. Wellness must also grow within the context of an ecological model that positions you in the world with other people in interpersonal relationships within institutional and community contexts.

If teaching is your talent, then you have an awesome responsibility to do it well—as in well-being and with wellness. In your calling to be a teacher, you also need to feel the calling into human relationships. A plaque on my desk reminds me that "words are the voice of the heart." Although words differentiate us from other life forms, this text broadens the scope of communication to include pictures, numbers, body language, rhythms, and environmental cues. Your ability to perceive the signs, symbols, and patterns of different communication elements will make educating for health more relational. I stated in *Multiple Intelligences: Different Ways to Educate for Health* (Ubbes, 2004):

> Perhaps your greatest challenge will be practicing multiple representations (more than one example) of how to communicate and educate for health in intelligent ways. Having this professional development will enable you to work with a diverse population of people with different needs, interests, preferences, abilities, and backgrounds in health, wellness, and prevention. Knowing one way to educate for health makes you a novice, but knowing multiple ways to educate for health will establish you as an expert. (p. 7)

## Relationships With People

People lie at the heart of teaching and learning. We can teach so many different topics, concepts, and skills in our fields and still not know the way to connect the information to the learner. The ability to connect information to the learner is called instructional design or pedagogy. No amount of instructional pedagogy will woo the learner if she does not connect to the heart of the communicator. The communicator can be a teacher, a speaker, a presenter, a facilitator, a parent, or an acquaintance. The deciding factor is *who* is interacting with *whom*? The message of the moment lies as background to that interaction.

There needs to be an interaction between teacher and learner in which the information that is communicated has an effect. That effect can be either positive or negative, but something must happen. If there is no resulting change, then the message did not matter.

A person gives off vibrations of energy that are positive, negative, or neutral. Analogous to a pebble that is dropped into water to initiate a ripple in a pond, a teacher can send a vibration that forms a ripple effect through his classroom. The first vibration must be felt by one or more people in order for their own perceptions to set up a wave of kinetic energy that moves additional people. If a child seems to have chaotic and random energy that is inappropriate for a place or space, the effective teacher or wise parent will help redirect the child's energy into a vibration more in flow with the needs of the majority. Although we rarely speak of children as being energetic vibrations, we can learn to direct their energy so they practice being attentive and focused. In middle school, the words and actions that preteens express are often moody, ranging from lows to highs, so even those vibrations must be attended to and redirected.

In the classroom, teachers often use props, books, and technologies to direct and redirect students' attention so they are better able to connect with the intended message of the lesson. Often these concrete tools for teaching are called hooks, doors, and entry points into the learning episode. These tools, empowered by the messages of the teacher, engage the multiple senses and intelligences of the students. When the learners see, hear, smell, sense, or touch a message, the experience is more likely to be memorable (and to be retained in emotional memory). Learning is much more interesting when two or more senses are engaged to provoke interest and novelty. We all have experienced learning something by seeing and hearing, but what if you include an additional sense to make the learning three-dimensional or more?

For example, if a parent tries to introduce a new food in an evening dinner, the child can hear, see, and taste the new food and even touch the texture of the food in the hand or mouth. Taste tests such as this are often done in supermarkets and even classrooms when a health teacher wants to increase the students' repertoire of fruits and vegetables. Whenever the teacher moves off the center stage for learning—known as "a sage on the stage"—into the role of "a guide on the side," children have more opportunities to interact with the subject matter and make more lasting, memorable connections.

In the case of taste tests, Satter (1987) suggests it takes approximately seven times before a person likes a new food. How many parents and teachers give children and youth enough practice time to teach their senses to attend to something new? I believe learning that slows down to engage the human senses will have more wellness benefits. Effective educators select a variety of props and multisensory messages to provoke the learners' attention. Teachers who use provocative materials that appeal to the head, heart, and hands of students will establish a greater learning potential than teachers who use few materials, and those without care and reason.

Teachers and students can co-create the curriculum by negotiating the ebb and flow of positive, negative, and neutral vibrations. Teachers must have sensitivity toward reading human cues and mannerisms initiated by body language and a posture of open ears, eyes, and supportive senses. Effective teachers read not only the senses of their learners but also the contextual cues of time, place, and situations for a sense of appropriateness. If well rested, well hydrated, and well nourished, teachers will be sensitive and aware of slight variations in the patterned behaviors of others. If teachers have deficiencies in their basic health needs, then they will be able to attend only to these deficiencies. However, by practicing daily healthful habits of self-care, teachers are better able to attend to others in a more caring, competent, and transformative way. In short, the relationship you have with yourself plays an important role in how you attend to others in relationships with you.

## Plans for Reflective Practice

For co-creations in the curriculum to surface, the teacher must plan for a rhythm of quiet followed by activity or activity followed by quiet. An engaging curriculum is always one of balance—the yin and yang of tensions created by opposites that can be seen as complementary. The metaphor of a pond gives us additional insights into the dynamics of the teaching–learning process as well. The surface is one part of the whole pond, but the depths of the water can bring a hidden wholeness that engages the paradox of opposites, e.g., above and below or across and within.

When teaching my health education pedagogy courses, I ask my students to reflect on common readings in both oral and written forms. I provide students with several choices of readings for a particular health theme each week (e.g., social, intellectual, spiritual, physical, and emotional). They read their chosen articles outside of class to prepare for an in-class discussion with their colleagues (called a learning community). The purpose of the learning community is to talk with peers who have read the same article and to negotiate shared meaning through dialogue and discussion.

Table 7.1 shows the comparisons between dialogue, discussion, and debate along the 5 D continuum of closed to open communication. The

Table 7.1　**The 5 D Continuum: Closed to Open Communication**

| Didactic | Discipline | Debate | Discussion | Dialogue |
|---|---|---|---|---|
| To tell and teach | To correct and redirect | To take sides on the information | To make your point | To honor another's voice and perspective |

Closed, one-way communication ————————————————→ Open, two-way communication

Talking ————————————————————————→ Talking and listening

purpose of dialogue is to reach understanding by honoring another's voice and perspective. The purpose of discussion is to make your point. And the purpose of debate is to argue successfully for your position over that of an opponent. Since my goal for learning communities is to establish weekly opportunities for reflective practice, I encourage the habits of mind of listening and speaking in the form of dialogue. During the third of four steps in learning communities, the students seek a "quiet and stillness" among the group members for 5 minutes. During this quiet time, the students think about a personal connection to the reading in a different way, now informed by other points of view from peers and from the professional expert who wrote the original source. This 5-minute time continues to challenge some students, who fidget in their seats as they attempt to make the time go away. After 5 minutes, I ask them to write in their learning journals for 10 minutes about the shared reading experiences. During their writing segment, students move into a discussion with themselves on paper.

One of the reasons I structure this oral and written reflection time into my course is that many university students are still learning how to think and talk about professional principles and practices. Writing is an excellent way to capture your thinking as a segue into oral re-tellings. As you gain in expertise, you will need increasing time to extend and add to the story lines of other professionals. Sometimes you may end up debating a particular principle or practice of your work when you socialize with those in your profession. However, because debates are objective, fact-proving exercises that often manipulate the ideas of people for personal gain, I do not often use debates when educating for health. There are plenty of assignments such as research papers or grant proposals that require the citing of evidence for a particular cause, issue, or problem, a skill that should be developed by all professionals. But there is a greater need for adequate time and space for reflection on pedagogical principles and practices, which encourage deeper meanings to emerge. In the end, if you know content details on the five habits of health and can model the five habits of mind, you will model an elementary understanding of the teaching–learning process in health education. How the habits of health and habits of mind are integrated into real-life examples in school, home, and community contexts becomes an important journey of expertise. However, the final test may be whether you can craft lessons that compel your learners to access and use valid information in one or more ways so that each learner can make his or her own cognitive-behavioral connections for improving personal health and well-being. Ultimately, it is up to each learner to convert egocentric learning into making a difference in the world, using his or her gifts and talents.

Throughout your career, I encourage you to sit and reflect on new information in relation to what you already know. Integrating new information with prior knowledge requires you to negotiate change through the concept pair of stability and adaptability. Note that the word *ability* is found in both stability and adaptability, so a teacher must have the ability to be a change agent and to be stable in an unpredictably changing world. As an agent of change, you will be more successful if you help young people recognize, understand, and appreciate their own abilities to negotiate change. We can turn to a picture book called *A Quiet Place* by Douglas Wood (2002) to help us with this challenge. The story line reminds the reader that "sometimes a person needs a quiet place." Although an academic classroom is often far from a comfortable place for reflection, Wood offers an overview of possibilities for many quiet places as you retreat from chaos. Here are his suggestions:

> A place to rest your ears from bells ringing, . . . grown-ups talking and radios playing. . . . The woods could be your quiet place. . . . The beach could be your quiet place. . . . The desert could be your quiet place. . . . A pond could be your quiet place. . . . A cave could be your quiet place. . . . A hilltop could be your quiet place. . . . A snowdrift could be your quiet place. . . . A museum could be your quiet place. . . . A library could be your quiet place. . . . You could come home and clean your room and read your own books and think your own thoughts and feel your own feelings and discover the very best quiet place of all—the one that's always there, no matter where you go or where you stay—the one inside of you. (pp. 3-24)

## Contextual Issues of Space and Place

I try to honor individual differences with respect to reflection. I watch for signs and cues from students who really love the experience and from those who often have disdain for quiet thinking. In the professional preparation of teachers and health educators, I know we must honor the needs and interests of all who wish to teach. However, reflection is a skill that you must learn in order to be an effective and competent educator of health. You don't have to like reflection, but you will need to respect it, because in so doing, you are respecting who you are and who you are becoming. The frequency and duration of time given to reflective practice will reward you with personal meaning making, understanding, and, eventually, wisdom.

Knowing how you learn and why a particular strategy or activity feels engaging or uncomfortable allows you to negotiate and plan learning experiences for others. I call this teaching from your strengths and learning through your weaknesses. When planning and implementing lessons for others, you will teach *inside* your comfort zone, but you should also be willing to step *outside* your comfort zone for your learners. This directional advice of inside and outside your comfort zone can be understood by the analogy of living inside and outside a box. Of course, the box could represent your home or residence, your personal boundary or frame of reference, or your risk-taking preferences. I have been teaching for several decades, so my understanding of the box is represented by a variety of images and metaphors. The challenge, of course, is that all teachers must negotiate a comfort zone that is dynamic and flexible for self and others.

Relationships are explained by Gardner's theory of multiple intelligences through his focus on the intrapersonal (self) and interpersonal (others). Gardner (1999) does not expect us to design lessons with all eight intelligences in mind; nor does he admire teachers who get several intelligences into one lesson, thereby claiming success for many ways of knowing. Instead, Gardner encourages us to think of entry points into a lesson (i.e., like an open door), selecting from a variety of options to introduce the subject matter. I believe that learners need to practice multiple symbol systems, for example semiotics, to gain access to information. The more we use a variety of words, pictures, numbers, rhythms, body languages, and environmental cues to educate for health, the more likely our learners will gain access to and recognize the different channels and forms of health-promoting messages. However, understanding health-related messages is more than recognizing multiple signs, symbols, and patterns in information. We must help young people to be intelligent in employing their cognitive-behavioral abilities—that is, habits of health and habits of mind—in multiple contexts, leading to a higher quality of life. Of course, they must also be able to recognize the harmful cues to action that lead to high-risk, compromising lifestyles.

Ellison (2001) extends Gardner's work by her own exploration of the personal intelligences, suggesting we need to move between the intrapersonal and interpersonal intelligences when planning our lessons. I often refer to these two intelligences as intrapersonal/introspective (I/I) and interpersonal/social (I/S) because they help us understand the contrast between being alone in quiet and being together in active engagement with people. Our comfort zones in moving between the intrapersonal and interpersonal intelligences help students practice interactions with self and others. Although children and adolescents operate out of an egocentric point of view, we should be moving children into and out of their comfort zones into building an awareness of and involvement with community. We can start with the practice of "still waters run deep," but I encourage balancing that exercise with the practice of finding common pathways that move people of all ages and backgrounds into the wisdom of "a river runs through us." Using this metaphor, I now turn inward to a discussion about health.

## A River Runs Through You

"A river runs through you" can serve as imagery for your cardiovascular system and its extensive network of blood vessels, which stretch through your body for miles. There are two main types of blood vessels that carry blood. Veins carry blood that travels toward your heart, and arteries carry blood that travels away from your heart. Blood runs through your arteries and veins to supply nutrients (e.g., carbohydrates) to your muscles so they can contract and relax as they move your body. The heart, a special cardiac muscle, will beat for you 100,000 times each day, every day while you are living. Each heartbeat lets you know that you are getting a steady supply of blood and nutrients to sustain your life.

Your blood is made up of important fluids that resemble a river. Many streams have clear and free-moving water that originates in rivers, lakes, or springs. Water, plasma, and blood cells are the parts of your blood that flow into and out of your heart.

Occasionally, your river of blood can be stopped by debris and logjams that impede the river's flow. When this happens inside the blood vessel, we say the artery is occluded, or blocked. When this happens in a blood vessel leading toward the heart, a heart attack occurs. When blockage happens in an artery leading toward the brain, a stroke occurs.

Your heart is an organ that symbolizes love and life. We can explain this from a wellness perspective to give this symbolism deeper meaning. In social health, we care and feel an attraction for other people, leading us into friendship and even intimacy. If those people are in our families or close circle of friends, we have a deeper commitment of care known as love. In emotional health, love is known as the ultimate in human feelings. Loving feelings are characterized by supportive and accepting expressions of care (not rejecting comments and actions) that humans consciously choose to offer. Feelings are also embedded in cultural nuances and contexts. In contrast, emotions are often characterized by physiological responses to life that are common across all people (e.g., fear, joy, depression, anger, shame). Because of their neurobiological nature, emotions often occur subconsciously (i.e., below our conscious awareness). When educating for health, we can teach young people to recognize the signs and signals of human emotions via body language so they can negotiate their personal problems of stress and conflict. This body-language approach opens the door for additional elements of language, which integrates words, pictures, numbers, rhythms, and environmental cues for managing their stress and conflict.

In physical health, the blood circulates through the body and heart, giving us our source of life. Without a heart and blood, we would not have a physical existence; we would not be alive. In spiritual health, the source of life may be a higher power that makes your life meaningful—often symbolized by love and captured by the soul. Depending on the religious traditions found among people who worship in churches, synagogues, or mosques, to name a few, blood can also mean sacrificial love. In the wellness model, spiritual health does not need to have its meaning in religion because each of us has a spirit. Hawks, Hull, Thalman, & Richins (1995) define spiritual well-being as a sense of relatedness or connectedness to another or others; a provision for meaning and purpose in life; an overall well-being to buffer stress, conflict, and energy; and a belief in and relationship with a power, entity, deity, or being higher than self. In intellectual health, we can sometimes talk about our passions and focused commitments to projects, careers, or events. Our ability to stay focused and committed to those passions requires reasoned thought that is informed by our emotions and feelings.

Many have written about the heart and soul of teaching. The heart of teaching may be found in the relationships you form with people who are willing or not willing to learn. There are relationships between people, relationships between people and their ideas, and relationships between people and their things. When educating for health, I believe human relationships matter most.

# Relationships Matter

What happens when a person comes through your classroom door? Or when you enter through the door of a building? Are you greeted? Are you made to feel welcome, or are you treated as a silent bystander? How do children get attended to? What happens when an adult comes through the door? As an interesting exercise, you might answer these questions in the context of your home, apartment, or dormitory room. You can also compare and contrast the different experiences you have as you enter and leave classrooms each day on your college campus.

Given (2002) reports on a Purdue University experiment cited in Ackerman (1990), in which

> a librarian brushed the hands of half the students as they checked out books. On leaving the library, the investigators asked the students several questions about their satisfaction with the library services. Those whose hands were physically touched reported significantly higher levels of satisfaction with the library—and life in general—than those not touched. They rated the librarian friendlier, but they were unaware that they had been touched. As subtle as this small gesture was, it clearly demonstrates the effect of touch on adults. (p. 89)

In the classroom, we could translate that study into some basic greetings: May I shake your hand? Pat you on the back? Give you a hug? Give you a high five? Depending on the familiarity you have with your students and the level of trust you sense between each student and you, you may not need to ask for permission for each of these greetings. However, the point is that human interaction affects your students' satisfaction with life (and learning) and is highly dependent on your willingness to open your heart to another person.

As you let people into your life, what do they find? How does the door to your heart operate? Open or closed? Free or barred? Renewed or bruised? Softened or hardened by the changes of life? Do you know people who have a heart of stone? Who do not warm up to you even after you greet them with a smile, or a handshake, or a pleasant greeting of invitation? Children or grown-ups who demonstrate a cold disposition are said to have a hardened heart. A hardened heart is like a tablet of stone on which a story of fear, addiction, hopelessness, or disconnect is written. Even though we all have enemies that prevent us from experiencing freedom from want and fear, we must also learn to face our feelings and not shut down or shut out the possibilities of living a life of potential.

Imagine one of your students who rarely seems happy. Perhaps he is distant and paralyzed by an external pressure that only he can know. Beneath a hard protective shell that seems impenetrable, you notice how harshly and rudely the child reacts to you and others. You may want to connect with that student but not be able to find the right access point beyond the cold shoulder, the hardened look, or closed body posture that speaks to the pain inside. The natural reaction for most people is to play the same game of disconnect and move on to someone who appreciates the care and concern you have to offer. However, teachers are called to a higher level of relationships in which they demonstrate a caring and compassionate heart no matter what. You don't have to sell your own soul on a daily basis, but it is wise to try—and then try again when the spirit moves you. Sometimes we understand this when a child is overly rambunctious or rebellious. Parents would say the child has a strong will; teachers might say the child is mean spirited.

Relationships do matter. Until a teacher and a student have generated a relationship of trust, there is less chance for individual freedoms in the classroom. Human interactions need freedom to be; freedom to express; freedom to change; and freedom to face one's deepest feelings in a very private sense without fear of rejection, ignorance, or conformity. Pain may be universal, but we need not assume one size fits all. No two people experience an event or situation in exactly the same way. Too often, teachers are eager to say, "I know what you mean," or "I had that happen to me once," or "I know how you feel." These generalizations need to be withheld until you have created a space for individual affirmation. A compassionate response is to validate and accept the student for her feelings, facial expressions, and mannerisms, including spoken words. Sometimes that means identifying and naming feelings for the student to adopt or asking open-ended questions that help her articulate her ideas.

Our role as teachers is not to change the person or move him to a new place because it worked for us or for someone else. As teachers, we can diagnose and identify a response that is unique for that individual based on the multitude of available options. (See figure 1.4 on pages 14 through 16 and tables 3.2 and 3.3 on pages 69 and 70, respectively.) Our role is to guide the student to a variety of available choices on a continuum of good, better, best—including laying out the consequences if he continues to make inappropriate or less than ideal choices. A teacher who is caring and compassionate will take the time to uncover the hardships that limit the student, creating a place and space for helping the student face his feelings.

We cannot truly know another's depth of pain or joy, but we can learn to reflect feelings back to the person with care. That includes the complexity of "double-dip" feelings, which surface in our changing facial expressions and mannerisms. Double-dip feelings, or having two feelings occur simultaneously for the same situation or event, remind us how we might be happy yet sad about moving to a new school, excited yet afraid by the start of a new class, and confused yet relieved when solving a problem. These moments of conflicting emotions take time to process and understand. A caring and compassionate teacher will slow the pace of expectations so that the student can invest in her own discovery.

Each of us wishes to be seen, heard, understood, and touched by tenderness. When there is continued harshness or hardening of the heart, we can maybe understand why students choose rejection, ignorance, and stubbornness. Many students know how it feels to be disconnected from their basic needs and to want something as simple as acceptance and validation from peers and caregivers. We don't have to like the behaviors, but we need to validate each student as a person who has value and worth no matter what. The harshness of breaking the law may suggest a different set of circumstances. But even in the discomfort of mistakes and in the violation of rules and regulations, a student can learn to face her feelings in a mirror, in a reflective pond, or in the caring friendship of another's face. Many times, the unmet needs of a student are expressed through anger, an emotion that needs a compassionate response, which is rarely given. Often, fear is the emotion that underlies so many of our worries and concerns. As an emotional burst of anger emerges, we need to watch for the behavioral style of aggression toward self and others.

In summary, facing our feelings can be hard work. Perhaps we face our most difficult feelings through stories written in books, as screenplays, as theatrical productions, or as works of art. In the end, the personal story surfaces from the fabric of the inspired work, and we gain meaning and insights from those connections. By paying attention to how the words and feelings touch our hearts, we gain access to our own souls and learn to uncover the enemies of the heart. As our feelings surface, quite often in raw reality, we must be willing to expose the truths of our own experiences. The truth can set one free. However, when a truth is shared without validation, a journey is stopped for the moment until the person decides what to do. No amount of learning can take place until the person learns from himself. That is what makes learning with integrity so powerful in our quest as educators. Until we have attempted this work in our own life, it will continue to masquerade as a barrier to teaching and learning.

During our attempts to help a student, we may feel guarded and protective of our own character so as not to be wounded in our moments of generosity. This is where we truly learn to be a teacher (or a parent or a guardian) to young people. We can learn to dedicate our lives to teaching people first and our subject matter second.

## Informed Learning Episodes

Information sharing between teacher and students is optimal when they are eye to eye and face to face. Without this posturing, much of what the teacher offers will be rejected, discarded, or ignored because it lacks relevance for the learner. One might argue that the student loses out, and it is his responsibility to get the job of learning done, but the student must experience a connection to the teacher *and* the subject matter for full engagement to occur. Schooling is replete with learners who have experienced one without the other, although both can be embraced hand in hand. The novice teacher may choose to focus on teaching the subject matter at the expense of other options, but such an approach only distances a student's experience from that of the teacher. As you both struggle to cover new ground in understanding your individual journeys, a cooperative respect is formed.

Teaching and learning require a give and take of needs and interests between teacher and students. Too often, grown-ups are the sole decision makers in the classroom. Progressive teachers soon learn that child-centered classrooms need to be balanced with the structure of teacher-directed classrooms. This is what curriculum theorists call the co-curriculum. If you have not had a university experience that leaves space for your interpretations and inquiry-based practices as a novice teacher, then your professional development will not serve you well in places where you are expected to solve problems with more than yesterday's tools and technologies. A dynamic professional who educates for health and well-being must be able to solve problems and craft plans, products, and performances that lead to a quality of life for all learners.

## Professional Practices That Support a Relational Pedagogy: We Need Each Other

Human relationships are at the heart of instructional design. When educating for health, try to focus on the relationship between people and their ideas in order to inform others and, ultimately, transform the world. Communication is created through different signs, symbols, and patterns of information. By studying the basic elements of communication and the 5 D continuum of closed to open communication (table 7.1), we can help young people access information that is connected to their lives. We can also honor different styles of communication when we seek to build a relational pedagogy with our learners.

Relational pedagogy means that human relationships are the pathways to teaching and learning. Greenfield (1984) suggests that people whose relationships tend to be shallow are usually uninvolved in other people's problems and retain a rather self-centered lifestyle. They are not people helpers; they can even be people avoiders. Some symptoms of superficial relationships include loneliness, insecurity, emptiness, faultfinding, psychosomatic illnesses, and self-centeredness. Greenfield continues:

> Just as our physical bodies suffer from a nutritional deficiency when we do not consume adequate amounts of vitamins, minerals, and various nutrients, so will our personalities suffer from a relational deficiency when we do not consume the support that comes from meaningful relationships. A hungry body will send out danger signals called hunger pains and eventually a neglected body will produce signs of illness and disease (dis-ease). Likewise, a deprived spirit will give out its danger signals: negative, critical, judgmental words and behavior. The person who complains a lot is telling us that he has a relational deficiency. All of us need to recognize that we "will find relational sufficiency only at the deeper levels" of our interpersonal relationships. (pp. 30-31)

As shown in figure 7.1, Greenfield has identified eight levels of relating. When people remain at level 5, relational deficiency develops, resulting in an unhappy, critical, complaining, and judgmental attitude. Relational sufficiency can be found at the deeper levels of 6, 7, and 8. When moving from level 1 toward level 8, one moves from secondary to primary relationships. Sociologists describe primary relationships as close, intimate, intense, personal, long-standing, and influential on one's growth and development. Secondary relationships are distant, impersonal, structured, utilitarian, short-lived, and not very influential on one's personality or behavior.

Relationships with your students and colleagues will move up and down the relationship levels of 1 to 7 but should not reach level 8 at any time while in your professional role. Sometimes a teacher or coach may be the parent of a student in the school, or occasionally an older brother or sister may teach a younger sibling or relative. You may even be aware of teachers in the same school who are married, unless the district has a policy against that. In any respect, level 8 intimacies do not belong in a professional workplace.

## Relationships Take Work

Relationships are a lot of work. As teachers, we are committed to developing good working relationships with students, colleagues, administrators, and parents. We need to value relationships with people and know

# Levels of Relating in Communication

### Level 1: The Avoidance Level

We pass people on the street or in the halls of a building. We avoid these people unintentionally.

### Level 2: The Greeting Level

We acknowledge each other with some kind of greeting: a spoken hello, a smile, or a nod.

### Level 3: The Separate Interests Level

We begin to probe to see if perchance we have some common interests. If our backgrounds, experiences, and tastes are sufficiently different, then our conversations will tend to reach a dead end.

### Level 4: The Common Interests Level

If we discover that we have some common interests, then our relationship will probably deepen. At this level, people merely share ideas in the search for friendship, but feelings are not a major part of the relationship.

### Level 5: The Social Interaction Level

Our common interests provide the opportunity to share these activities beyond the conversational stage. Social interaction means that two or more people engage in a common activity.

### Level 6: The Caring Level

Moving from level 5 to level 6 is a major step in any relationship. To care means to listen, to learn, to reach out, and to make yourself available. Caring produces depth and closeness.

### Level 7: The Sharing Level

The sharing level is where you open up, become vulnerable, run some risks, and reveal the true and honest you. People with whom you can share your inner self are people who will reciprocate. Relationships at this level provide us with mirrors that allow us to see ourselves and help others close to us see themselves. We really can't find ourselves without other people.

### Level 8: The Intimacy Level

Intimacy takes time and commitment, so there will be very few to whom we will relate on this level in our entire lifetimes. This level of relating is the deepest level of all and includes verbal and nonverbal, physical and nonphysical, and emotional and spiritual interactions.

**Figure 7.1**  Levels of relating in communication.

Reprinted, by permission, from G. Greenfield, 1984, *We need each other* (Grand Rapids, MI: Baker Publishing Group), 26-28.

that relationships with others do matter in teaching and learning. We should also not lose sight of the relationships we have with our own family members and friends outside the workplace. Sometimes teachers put so much time into their jobs that they do not have enough energy to work on relationships at home. Other teachers are so distracted by the demands of personal and family relationships away from school that they cannot adequately build the type of teacher–student relationships that are necessary for effective learning.

## Role of Schools in Building a Safe and Supportive Environment for Learning

Schools need to build safe and supportive environments for learning so that students open up and make natural connections to people and their ideas. When kids make mistakes, having caring supports and clear boundaries in place lets them learn and relearn how to behave and how to respond to situations. Emotional outbursts, withdrawn hibernations, and feelings in between these two extremes are possible responses when kids experience change and chaos in their lives. Helping kids express their feelings in appropriate ways is one part of our role in educating for health. This involves developing a feelings vocabulary and practicing conflict resolution and stress management skills. Many ideas for effective communication and conflict resolution are shared throughout this book.

When we focus on the expressed needs of kids, we may not totally understand their underlying motivations or intentions. In fact, *what* you see and hear may not be what they *meant* to do or say. Sometimes middle school kids will even misread the physical and emotional cues of others. Children with autism are unable to accurately read the faces of their caregivers. There are many adults, including well-meaning parents, who take kids at face value and miss the opportunities for building deeper relationships beneath the surface of bodily and facial expressions.

I have learned that human nature is constantly changing. I have observed (sometimes in frustration) that the response a child or adolescent gives me in one situation may not be the same intended response in the next situation. It's like a disconnect between what they say and what they mean or what they say and what they do. This proclivity to give mixed messages is developmentally normal, and it takes a great deal of patience and tolerance to know when to overlook these experiments in communication. When a pattern begins to emerge, however, teachers, parents, and caregivers must be able to give feedback to cue a more appropriate response next time . . . and the next time . . . and the next time!

When you take the time to be healthy yourself, leading to greater security and stability in who you are and what you need, it becomes easier to respond to others. Teachers do not need to be saints in this regard, but you do need to recognize the reciprocal and changing nature of social and emotional health. Conflicts arise when our needs and wants (interests) are not in alignment with the needs and wants (interests) of others. When we move into debates and discussions, conflict may escalate until at least one person is willing to adjust her position to resolve the situation through a posture of dialogue (see table 7.1).

In your classroom, how do you imagine dealing with personal conflicts with a student or a colleague? Nepo (2005) cautions that "in a moment of being more concerned with the task than the person doing it, we slip out of compassion" (p. 156). This can easily happen in lessons where the assignments to be completed are the objects of our focus instead of the person who is doing the learning (or not learning because of a life distraction, real or perceived). In what way does this help you understand the truths of teaching? And the truths of your own life?

None of us will be able to effectively educate for health if we focus mostly on the five fruits and vegetables or the three glasses of milk instead of on the human relationship that needs our compassion. Such compassion may mean that we offer our encouraging support or no support at all so the child can learn the hard way. But the realities are grim when the child's consistent patterns are lacking in habits of health and underdeveloped in habits of mind.

Nepo also speaks of our adult tendencies in establishing relationships:

> When a relationship is changing—that is, birthing or dying—and we deny the pain of that truth, we often thrust ourselves into a side life of denial, whereby we solicit misadventures, such as affairs or other addictions, to soothe the ache we carry rather than face things as they are. And yet an opposite response to the same situation can mire us in a painful journey of indulgence, whereby we endlessly process and circle the dysfunctions we've created rather than accept things as they are and repair or move on. (p. 220)

In the end, the acceptance of self and the courage to grow and change remain the true challenges of a life worth living. When we relate to another human being with the compassion to show love and acceptance for who he is, first and foremost, then that person gains more freedom to risk the next steps of what he does to engage in habits of health and habits of mind.

This text targets professionals like you who are called to be caring, competent, and transformative with young people. You will experience effective teaching and learning practices when you develop a reflective philosophy integrated with a pedagogy grounded in intrapersonal theories (e.g., multiple intelligences, learning styles, and constructivism) and evidence-based instructional strategies (EBIS).

## CHAPTER FEATURES

### Principles of Practice

- The metastory of life is how to bridge people and their ideas to make the world a better place so that individuals and communities have a higher quality of life.

- When educating for health, give young people access to their own stories so they can form their identities as physical beings, social beings, intellectual beings, emotional beings, and spiritual beings. These multiple dimensions of health form us into human beings.

- Learning communities are a way to develop relationships between people and their ideas. Professionals who know and practice the different forms of discourse (i.e., didactic, discipline, debate, discussion, and dialogue) will increase their competence in a relational pedagogy.

- Relationships matter when you educate for health. Professionals who are committed to practicing a relational pedagogy honor human relationships as the pathways to teaching and learning.

- Your professional identity of who you are (chapter 1), ways to be (chapter 2), ways to think (chapter 3), and ways to know (chapter 4) is foundational to how you structure your personal and professional stories (chapter 5) and how you design lessons using evidence-based instructional strategies (EBIS) as a pedagogical framework (chapter 6). Ultimately, how you build relationships with yourself and others (chapter 7) is the pathway to understanding and wisdom.

### Teacher Voices

The following was written by an undergraduate student enrolled in a health education pedagogy class.

As future teachers, it is very important that we not only learn how to teach students but also that we become acquainted and understanding of their personal lives. I feel that although teachers are given the entire day to influence a child, perhaps the most influential part of the day comes when they face the outside world. Therefore, I feel it is my responsibility to create a classroom atmosphere in which students are comfortable and excited to learn. I think that one way to help deal with "outside problems" is to maybe have a system where each day when the students walk into the classroom they can write a statement about how they feel or they can write something that is simply on their mind. This would give them a chance to release some stress and also allow me to become more aware of the situations in their lives. For example, they could write, "I only got two hours of sleep last night" or "I'm fighting with my mom." Does anyone think this is a good idea? I pretty much just pulled it out of nowhere.

*Carolyn Stewart Schutte, Miami University alumna in health education, 1999.*

## Seeds of Growth:
## Signs, Symbols, and Patterns of Living and Learning

In chapter 3, you learned about automatic negative thinking (ANT) that compromises our cognitive-emotional identities (table 3.2) as well as some cognitive-emotional "bugs" (table 3.3). See table 7.2 for a comparison. When educating for health, it is important to manage your ineffective and negative thinking patterns by recognizing them in your daily thinking and asking others to support you in reducing them. The metaphor of bugs and the acronym of ANT (automatic negative thinking) can help you catch some of these active pests in your social-cognitive environment. One pest at a party or picnic is not too bad. But too many pests will spoil the fun for you and others.

Table 7.2 **Bugs Versus ANTs**

| Bugs (ways we bug our brains to be ineffective) | ANTs (ways we carry negative weight around) |
|---|---|
| Mind reader (clairvoyant) bug | Mind reader thinking |
| Blame (not my fault) bug | Blame thinking |
| Invalidator (negative shadow) bug | Focus on the negative thinking |
| Perfection (shame and humiliation) bug | Guilt beating thinking |
| Past (might have been) bug | Guilt beating and all or nothing thinking |
| Future (worry and anxious) bug | Fortune telling thinking and feeling |
| Should (condemnation) bug | Guilt beating thinking |
| Magnifier (exaggerator) bug | Always thinking |

Source column 1: Equipping Ministries International (2000); source column 2: Amen, D. (2001).

In your learning journal, reflect on and write about the following questions:

- How will you break the habit of an ANT or bug in your life?
- How do you plan to help young people when you see or hear an ANT or bug running or buzzing around you?
- How can you ACT with **A**utomatic **C**ompassionate **T**houghts to help youth with these ANTs or bugs?

*Take-home message (generalization)*. Plan to make ACTs part of the climate in your relationships. Remember that when we teach others, there is up to a 95% retention rate in learning. Peer education programs are based on this educational principle.

## Web Links for Living and Learning

Go online to the Children's Picture Book Database at Miami University (www. lib.muohio.edu/pictbks). Look for picture books in the health and medicine category that include themes of feelings. The database has more than 40 keywords for locating different feelings in story lines. Picture books can talk about a feeling directly or indirectly in words from the characters, show the body language of the character experiencing the feeling, and provoke a personal connection with the feeling when the reader interacts with the book. For teaching different feelings or emotions directly through picture books, use the Boolean search option on this site to find specific books that combine a feeling with a habit of mind (e.g., happiness and goal setting; sadness and conflict resolution; assertiveness and verbal communication).

## Books for Living and Learning

After reading the picture book *Double-Dip Feelings* by Barbara Cain (2004), create your own template for two pages in a similar picture book that will show how you have experienced two feelings at the same time. Work in a small group of three people to combine your pages into a minibook for sharing with your colleagues or students. Perhaps some of your colleagues can write pages for an early childhood audience, and others can write pages for a middle childhood audience.

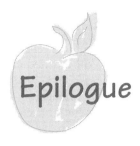

# Epilogue

In January 2005, the U.S. Surgeon General, the leader of the U.S. public health system, announced his agenda for "The Year of the Healthy Child." The public service announcement gave focus to "improving the body, mind, and spirit of the growing child," including the education of parents and caregivers on how to prevent negative health outcomes for children and youth.

This agenda was flanked by the Futures Initiative, the strategic development process of the U.S. Centers for Disease Control and Prevention (United States CDC, 2007b). In July 2004, the CDC aligned its priorities under two overarching health protection goals:

1. Preparedness: People in all communities will be protected from infectious, environmental, and terrorist threats.

2. Health promotion and prevention of disease, injury, and disability: All people will achieve their optimal life span with the best possible quality of health in every stage of life.

The CDC has also developed more targeted goals "to assure an improved impact on health at every stage of life, including infants and toddlers, children, adolescents, adults, and older adults" and "to help

> When we can connect to what lives both at the heart of our problems and at the heart of the problems of others, and listen to those connections, we become bridges to each other, the world, and to the spirit that informs everything. So, when we speak of integrity, we are speaking of how we care for the tender bridge between our innermost being and the common life of beings.
>
> © by Mark Nepo, *The Exquisite Risk: Daring to Live an Authentic Life*, 2005

ensure that all people are protected in safe and healthy communities so they can achieve their full life expectancy" (www.cdc.gov/od/oc/media/pressrel/r040513.htm).

As a new professional in education and health, you will need to be aware of national agendas such as the two just outlined so that you will be able to sense the impact that public health decisions may have on your work. You may not know how to read these patterns and trends until you have worked for a few years in schools and communities. Educators often learn about education messages from the U.S. Department of Education, whereas health professionals often learn about public health messages from the U.S. Department of Health and Human Services. Nonetheless, as a professional who will educate for health, you should learn about both of these departments of the federal government. You will also need to explore the challenges advanced by ideologies and policies that may seem to work at cross-purposes for human beings seeking a quality of life and learning.

As a progressive young professional, please learn to listen to, read, and talk about public health *and* education messages, then try to integrate them into your life's work. This conscious decision will be helpful for many people since you are responsible for both health and education initiatives, leading to health education. If you do not yet feel comfortable calling yourself a health educator (any more than you would feel comfortable calling yourself a physical educator or math educator), you might initially recognize your important responsibility for "educating for health." Only time will tell how committed you will become in this journey of health and wellness.

Even if every teacher in the United States knew how to teach health education to young people, there would still be gaps in teaching health-related information in schools. No one person can study and come to know both the education and health literatures in depth during an undergraduate education, but collectively we can share what we know to keep others informed. When you pursue a graduate degree, you will be required to know one body of literature thoroughly but also draw upon and be informed by multiple bodies of literature. These disciplinary and interdisciplinary stories are ways that other professionals have thought about and solved problems about education and health before you. Someday, you will contribute to that body of knowledge and possibly to the literature that is read and written by scholars and practitioners alike.

Unfortunately, in your undergraduate preparation, you may be required to take only one or two health courses (Ubbes, Cottrell, Ausherman et al., 1999). Conversely, health education majors may take only one or a few education courses. I continue to encourage education professionals to walk across the learning bridge called health promotion and disease prevention to meet with health professionals—who will walk across the learning bridge in education—in order to establish an education and health partnership. We must cross these bridges frequently to learn from one another. We must also invite others to take the journey with us. We do this boundary crossing on behalf of children and youth who are not fully aware of the reasons for disciplinary and cross-disciplinary stories.

The important result of this boundary crossing is that two major concepts—education and health—are joined to form the disciplinary story of health education. On the education side of the story, you know disciplinary stories from your preK-12 experiences in science, social studies, mathematics, language arts, music, physical education, art, and health education. There are also cross-disciplinary stories from your university course work: educational leadership, educational psychology, and teacher education, to name a few. I know that health issues and concepts can serve as important content knowledge in many of your education courses, from which you will subsequently weave your personal stories and professional theories in your work with young people.

We still need more creative and flexible ways to give professionals access to interdisciplinary course work and experiences in schools and universities in the United States. This requires a concerted effort by teachers and faculty who will cross boundaries and be risk takers to show how health is foundational to the curriculum of life. Promoting health through the interdisciplinary connections of topics, concepts, and skills will create a network of professionals who see how health serves as an infrastructure for who we are and how well we function as human beings. Ultimately, this professional network results when *all* people get access to skill development in health education courses, beginning in their formative years and extending across the bridge into higher education. Without consistent education about health, we cannot realize a higher quality of life for human beings.

With that goal in mind, I challenge you to teach health-related topics, concepts, and skills to all your students in traditional and progressive ways so that children and teens gain access and commitment to their own health and well-being. Regardless of the professional careers your students choose in the future, a changing continuum of wellness and illness will intersect their private, personal, and professional lives.

To date, health educators have not done an adequate job of naming and framing the health-related topics, concepts, and skills that other disciplinary experts might adopt for our collaborative work. Although many people have blundered through this by trial and error with limited *formal* course work in preK-12 health education, I believe our unique stories and professional theories are often interwoven to educate for health—for better or for worse. This book purposely leaves space for interpretations on all sides of this issue, from laypersons to professionals, so we can journey toward the ultimate goal: to know and do our part in increasing the quality of life for human beings and to make a difference in the world. Since each of us has something to offer the curriculum of life, may your own journey help inform others of this awesome possibility.

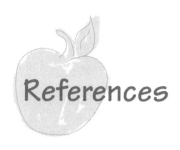

# References

Ackerman, D. (1990). *A natural history of the senses.* New York: Vintage Books.

Agassi, M. (2002). *Hands are not for hitting.* Minneapolis: Free Spirit.

Agassi, M. (2004). *Words are not for hurting.* Minneapolis: Free Spirit.

Allegrante, J.P., & Sleet, D.A. (Eds.). (2004). *Derryberry's educating for health: A foundation for contemporary health education practice.* San Francisco: Jossey-Bass.

Amen, D.G. (1997). *Mindcoach for kids: Teaching kids and teens to think positive and feel good.* Fairfield, CA: Mind Works Press.

Angelo, T.A., & Cross, K.P. (1993). Classroom assessment techniques: A handbook for college teachers. San Francisco: Jossey-Bass.

Armstrong, T. (2003). *The multiple intelligences of reading and writing: Making the words come alive.* Alexandria, VA: Association for Supervision and Curriculum Development.

Berk, R.A. (2001). Using music with demonstrations to trigger laughter and facilitate learning in multiple intelligences. *Journal on Excellence in College Teaching, 12*(1), 87-107.

Berman, M., & Brown, D. (2000). *The power of metaphor: Story telling and guided journeys for teachers, trainers, & therapists.* Wales, UK: Crown House Publishing Limited.

Blumenfeld-Jones, D. (2004). Aesthetics, curriculum leadership, and curriculum thinking. *Journal of Curriculum and Pedagogy, 1*(2): 56-60.

Blythe, T., & Gardner, H. (1990). A school for all intelligences. *Educational Leadership, 47*(7), 33-37.

Bobbitt, J.F. (1918). *The curriculum.* Boston: Houghton Mifflin.

Bonaguro, J.A. (1981). PRECEDE for wellness. *Journal of School Health, 51,* 501-506.

Boyer, E.L. (1983). *High school: A report on secondary education in America.* New York: Carnegie Foundation for the Advancement of Teaching.

Bredeson, P.V. (2003). *Designs for learning: A new architecture for professional development in schools.* Thousand Oaks, CA: Corwin Press.

Brooks, J.G., & Brooks, M.G. (1993). *In search of understanding: The case for constructivist classrooms.* Alexandria, VA: Association for Supervision and Curriculum Development.

Brooks, J.G. (2002). *Schooling for life.* Arlington, VA: Association for Supervision and Curriculum Development.

Brown, E. (2005). The good life: Seagate's hard driving CEO. *Forbes.* Retrieved from www.Forbes.com.

Bunting, C.E. (2004). Balancing the middle school. *The Clearinghouse: A Journal of Educational Strategies, Issues, and Ideas, 77*(4): 146-147.

Cain, B.S. (2004). *Double-dip feelings: Stories to help children understand emotions* (2nd ed.). Washington, DC: Magination Press.

Carpenter, B.S., & Langston, L.P. (2004). Engaging contemporary art students: Making meaning in a visual world. *Journal of Curriculum and Pedagogy, 1*(2), 74-78.

Connelly, F.M., & Clandinin, D.J. (1988). *Teachers as curriculum planners: Narratives of experience.* Columbia University: Teachers College Press.

Costa, A.L., & Lowery, L. (1989). *Techniques for teaching thinking.* Pacific Grove, CA: Midwest Publications.

Costa, A.L., and Kallick, B. (2000). *Assessing and reporting on habits of mind.* Alexandria, VA: Association for Supervision and Curriculum Development.

Cropley, A.J. (2001). *Creativity in education and learning: A guide for teachers and educators.* Abingdon, Oxon: Routledge Falmer.

Curtis, J.L., & Cornell, L. (2006). *Is there really a human race?* New York: Harper Collins.

Danielson, C. (1996). *Enhancing professional practice: A framework for teaching.* Arlington, VA: Association for Supervision and Curriculum Development.

Darling-Hammond, L., & Sikes, G. (Eds.). (1999). *Teaching as the learning profession.* San Francisco: Jossey-Bass.

Deline, J. (1991). Why . . . can't they get along? Developing cooperative skills through physical education. *Journal of Physical Education, Recreation and Dance, 62*(1): 21-26.

Dewey, J. (1902). *The child and the curriculum.* Chicago: University of Chicago Press.

Dewey, J. (1934). *Art as experience.* New York: Minton Balch.

Dobrin, S.I. (1997). *Constructing knowledges: The politics of theory-building and pedagogy in composition.* Albany: State University of New York Press.

Dreifus, C. (2001, October 31). A conversation with John McWhorter: How language came to be, and change. *The New York Times.* www.nytimes.com.

Duke, N.K. (2000). 3.6 minutes per day: The scarcity of informational texts in first grade. *Reading Research Quarterly, 35,* 202-224.

*Economist, The.* (December 23, 2006). Captain Kirk's revenge: Emotion is essential to human survival, pp. 4, 6-7.

Eddy, J.M., Donahue, R.E., Webster, R.D., & Bjornstad, E.K. (2002). Application of an ecological perspective in worksite health promotion: A review. *American Journal of Health Studies, 17*(4): 197-202.

Ehlert, L. (1997). *Hands.* San Diego: Harcourt Brace.

Eisner, E. (2004). How the arts inspire curriculum and pedagogy synergy: Artistry and pedagogy in curriculum. *Journal of Curriculum and Pedagogy, 1*(2): 15-16.

Ellison, L. (2001). *The personal intelligences: Promoting social and emotional learning.* Thousand Oaks, CA: Corwin Press.

Enz, B.J. (2003). The a b c's of family literacy. In A. DeBruin-Pareki & B. Krol-Sinclair (Eds.), *Family literacy: From theory to practice* (pp. 50-67). Newark, DE: International Reading Association.

Equipping Ministries International. (2000). Cognitive emotional bugs. www.equippingministries.org.

Erickson, H.L. (1998). *Concept-based curriculum and instruction: Teaching beyond the facts.* Thousand Oaks, CA: Corwin Press.

Ericsson, A. (2005). Recent advances in expertise research: A commentary on the contributions to the special issue. *Applied Cognitive Psychology, 19*(2): 233-241.

Erikson, E. (1950). *Childhood and society.* New York: Norton.

ETR Associates. (2002). Inquiry questions asked by youth. www.etr.org/recapp.

Fahlberg, L.L., & Fahlberg, L.A. (1997). Wellness reexamined: A cross cultural perspective. *American Journal of Health Studies, 13*(1), 8-16.

Fein, G.G. (1981). Pretend play in childhood: An integrative review. *Child Development,* 52, 1095-1118.

Fisher, B., & Medvic, E.F. (2003). *For reading out loud: Planning and practice.* Portsmouth, NH: Heinemann.

Flinders, D.J. (2004). How the arts inspire curriculum and pedagogy synergy. *Journal of Curriculum and Pedagogy, 1*(2): 71-74.

Friere, P., & Faundez, A. (1989). *Learning to question.* New York: Pantheon.

Gagnon, G.W., & Collay, M. (2006). *Constructing learning designs: Key questions for teaching to standards.* Thousand Oaks, CA: Corwin Press.

Gardner, H. (1983). *Frames of mind: The theory of multiple intelligences.* New York: Basic Books.

Gardner, H. (1985). *Frames of mind: The theory of multiple intelligences* (paperback edition). New York: Basic Books.

Gardner, H. (1993). *Multiple intelligences: The theory in practice.* New York: Basic Books.

Gardner, H. (1995). Expert performance: Its structure and acquisition: Comment. *American Psychologist, 50,* 802-803.

Gardner, H. (1997). *Extraordinary minds: Portraits of 4 exceptional individuals and an examination of our own extraordinariness.* New York: Basic Books.

Gardner, H. (1999). *Intelligence reframed: Multiple intelligences for the 21st century.* New York: Basic Books.

Geertz, C. (1973). Thick description: Toward an interpretive theory of culture. In *The interpretation of cultures: Selected essays* (pp. 3-30). New York: Basic Books.

Geertz, C. 1973. *Interpretations of culture.* New York: Basic Books.

Gillmore, M.R., Archibald, M.E., Morrison, D.M., Wilsdon, A., Wells, E.A., Hoppe, M.J., et al. (2002). Teen sexual behavior: Applicability of the theory of reasoned action. *Journal of Marriage and Family, 64,* 885-897.

Given, B.K. (2002). *Teaching to the brain's natural learning systems.* Alexandria, VA: Association for Supervision and Curriculum Development.

Goldish, M. (2003). *Made by hand.* New York: Newbridge Educational Publishing.

Green, L.W., & Kreuter, M.W. (2005). *Health program planning: An educational and ecological approach.* Boston: McGraw-Hill.

Greenberg, J.S. (1985). Health and wellness: A conceptual differentiation. *Journal of School Health, 55*(10), 403-406.

Greenfield, G. (1984). *We need each other.* Grand Rapids, MI: Baker.

Gregory, G., & Chapman, C. (2002). *Differentiated instructional strategies: One size doesn't fit all.* Thousand Oaks, CA: Corwin Press.

Hall, E.T. (1976). *Beyond culture.* Garden City, NY: Anchor Books.

Halpern, D.F., & Nummedal, S.G. (1995). Closing thoughts about helping students improve how they think. *Teaching of Psychology, 22*(1), 82-83.

Hanley, M.S. (2004). Born to form: The synergy of curriculum and pedagogy through the arts. *Journal of Curriculum and Pedagogy, 1*(2): 21-25.

Harwayne, S., & New York City Board of Education. (2002). *Messages to ground zero: Children respond to September 11, 2001.* Portsmouth, NH: Heinemann.

Hawkins, J., & Blakeslee, S. (2004). *On intelligence.* New York: Henry Holt.

Hawks, S.R., Hull, M.L., Thalman, R.L., & Richins, P.M. (1995). Review of spiritual health: Definition, role, and intervention strategies in health promotion. *American Journal of Health Promotion, 9*(5), 371-378.

Haynes, J. (2007, August). Spotlight on English language learners: Giant steps: Writing workshops and English language learners. *Middle Ground,* 34-36.

Hillman, S.B. (1991). What developmental psychology has to say about early adolescence. *Middle School Journal,* September, 3-8.

hooks, b. (2004). *Skin again.* New York: Hyperion.

Hyerle, D. (2004). *Student successes with Thinking Maps®: School-based research, results, and models for achievement using visual tools.* Thousand Oaks, CA: Corwin Press.

Irwin, R.L. (2004). Unfolding aesthetic in/sights between curriculum and pedagogy. *Journal of Curriculum and Pedagogy, 1*(2): 43-51.

Janesick, V.J. (2004). Making connections: The reflective dialogue journal as a work of art to inspire and provide insight into curriculum and pedagogy. *Journal of Curriculum and Pedagogy, 1*(2): 56-60.

Joint Committee of the Association for the Advancement of Health Education and the American School Health Association. (1992). Health instruction responsibilities and competencies for elementary (K-6) classroom teachers. *Journal of Health Education, 23*(6): 352-353.

Joint Committee of the Association for the Advancement of Health Education, American School Health Association, National Middle School Association, American Association of School Administrators, and Council of Chief State School Officers. (1996). *Professional preparation standards for grades 4-9.* Reston, VA: AAHE.

Joint Committee on National Health Education Standards. (2007). *National health education standards: Achieving excellence.* Atlanta: American Cancer Society.

Jung, C. (1923). *Psychological types* (H.G. Baynes, Trans.). New York: Harcourt Brace.

Kind, S. (2004). Openings and undoings: The text of textiles in curriculum and pedagogy. *Journal of Curriculum and Pedagogy, 1*(2): 48-51.

King, A. (1995). Inquiring minds really do want to know: Using questioning to teach critical thinking. Special issue: Psychologists teach critical thinking. *Teaching of Psychology, 22*(1), 13-17.

Kreuter, M.W., & Wray, R.J. (2003). Tailored and targeted health communication: Strategies for enhancing information relevance. *American Journal of Health Behavior, 27*(Supplement 3), S227-S232.

Lasher, W. (2001, October). Warden's corner. *The Shamrock.* Lebanon, OH: St. Patrick's Episcopal Church.

Lazear, D. (1999). *Multiple intelligence approaches to assessment: Solving the assessment conundrum.* Tucson, AZ: Zephyr Press.

Lazear, D. (2003). *Eight ways of teaching: The artistry of teaching with multiple intelligences* (3rd ed.). Tucson, AZ: Zephyr Press.

Leamnson, R. (1999). *Thinking about teaching and learning: Developing habits of learning with first year college and university students.* Sterling, VA: Stylus Publishing.

Learning First Alliance. (2001). *Every child learning: Safe and supportive schools.* Baltimore: Association for Supervision and Curriculum Development.

Lerman, J. (2005). *101 best web sites for elementary teachers.* Eugene, OR: International Society for Technology in Education.

Lester, J. (2005). *Let's talk about race.* New York: HarperCollins.

Magolda, M.B. (2001). *Making their own way: Narratives for transforming higher education to promote self-development.* Sterling, VA: Stylus Publishing.

Magolda, M.B., & King, P.M. (Eds.). (2004). *Learning partnerships: Theory and models of practice to educate for self-authorship.* Sterling, VA: Stylus Publishing.

Malow-Iroff, M., Benhar, M., & Martin, S. (2005). Educational reform and the child with disabilities. In H. Johnson (Ed.), *Authentic educational reform.* New York: Erlbaum.

Martin, T. (1993). Turning points revisited: How effective middle-grades schools address developmental needs of young adolescent students. *Journal of Health Education Supplement,* November/December, S-24–S-27.

Marzano, R.J., Pickering, D.J., & Pollock, J.E. (2001). *Classroom instruction that works: Research-based strategies for increasing student achievement.* Alexandria, VA: Association for Supervision and Curriculum Development.

Marzano, R.J., Pickering, D.J., et al. (1997). *Dimensions of learning trainer's manual* (2nd ed.). Alexandria, VA: Association for Supervision and Curriculum Development.

McDermott, M. (2004). Curriculum lost/curriculum found: Theoretical wanderings. *Journal of Curriculum and Pedagogy, 1*(2): 66-70.

McLeroy, K.R., Bibeau, D., Steckler, A., & Glanz, K. (1988). An ecological perspective on health promotion programs. *Health Education Quarterly, 15,* 351-377.

McMillan, B., & Conner, M. (2003). Using the theory of planned behavior to understand alcohol and tobacco use in students. *Psychology, Health, & Medicine, 8*(3), 317-328.

Merton, T. (1989). Hagia sophia. In T.P. McDonnell (Ed.), *A Thomas Merton reader* (p. 506). New York: Doubleday.

Michigan Model for Health. www.emc.cmich.edu/mm/default.htm.

Montano, D.E., & Kasprzyk, D. (2002). The theory of reasoned action and the theory of planned behavior. In K. Glanz, K. Rimer, & F.M. Lewis (Eds.), *Health education and health behaviors: Theory, research, and practice,* 3rd ed. (pp. 67-98). San Francisco: Jossey-Bass.

Moran, S., Kornhaber, M., & Gardner, H. (2006). Orchestrating multiple intelligences: No need to create nine different lesson plans. Instead, design rich learning experiences that nurture each student's combination of intelligences. *Educational Leadership, 64*(1): 22-27.

Morris, A., & Heyman, K. (1998). *Tools.* New York: William Morrow.

Mullen, C.A. (2004). Curriculum and pedagogy synergy through the arts. *Journal of Curriculum and Pedagogy, 1*(2): 32-36.

Muth, Jon J. (2002). *The three questions: Based on a story by Leo Tolstoy.* New York: Scholastic.

National Commission for Health Education Credentialing (NCHEC). (1996). *A competency-based framework for professional development of certified health education specialists.* Allentown, PA: Author.

National Research Council. (2002). *How people learn: Bridging research and practice.* Washington, DC: National Academy Press.

Nepo, M. (2005). *The exquisite risk: Daring to live an authentic life.* New York: Three Rivers Press. www.MarkNepo.com

Newell, A., & Simon, H.A. (1972). *Human problem solving.* Englewood Cliffs, NJ: Prentice-Hall.

*NY Public Library Desk Reference.* (1989). New York: Simon & Schuster.

Nygard, B., & Koonce, S. (2002). *When Cody became a mouse potato.* Dubuque, IA: Kendall/Hunt.

Palmer, P.J. (1998). *The courage to teach: Exploring the inner landscape of a teacher's life.* San Francisco: Jossey-Bass.

Paratore, C. (2004). *26 big things small hands do.* Minneapolis: Free Spirit.

Parry, T., & Gregory, G. (1998). *Designing brain compatible learning.* Arlington Heights, IL: IRI SkyLight Professional Development.

Partnership for Clear Health Communication & Ask Me 3. (2003). *Tips for clear healthcare communication.* Retrieved from www.askme3.org.

Paul, R. (1999). *Critical thinking: Basic theories and structures.* Sonoma, CA: Foundation for Critical Thinking.

Perkins, D., & Blythe, T. (1994). Putting understanding up front. *Educational Leadership, 51*(5).

Perkins, D.N. (1986). *Knowledge as design.* Hillsdale, NJ: Erlbaum.

Piaget, J. (1954). *The construction of reality in the child.* New York: Basic Books.

Piaget, J. (1983). *Piaget's theory.* In P. Mussen (Ed.), *Handbook of child psychology,* 4th ed., vol. 1. New York: Wiley.

Pinar, W.F., Reynolds, W.M., Slattery, P., & Taubman, P.M. (1995). *Understanding curriculum: An introduction to the study of historical and contemporary curriculum discourses.* New York: Peter Lang.

Postman, N. (1995). The *end of education: Redefining the value of school.* New York: Vintage Books.

Prior, J.O., & Gerard, M.R. (2004). *Environmental print in the classroom: Meaningful connections for learning to read.* New York: International Reading Association.

Prochaska, J.O., & DiClemente, C.C. (1983). Stages and processes of self-change in smoking: Towards an integrated model of change. *Journal of Consulting Clinical Psychology, 51,* 390-395.

Ramachandran, V.S., & Oberman, L.M. (2006). Broken mirrors: A theory of autism. *Scientific American, 295*(5), 62-69.

Sallis, J.F., & Owen, N. (1997). Ecological models. In K. Glanz, F.M. Lewis, & B.K. Rimer (Eds.), *Health behavior and health education: Theory, research, and practice* (2nd ed.) (pp. 403-424). San Francisco: Jossey-Bass.

Sanchez, R. (1994). David Bleich and the politics of anti-intellectualism: A response. *Journal of Advanced Composition, 14,* 579-581.

Satter, E. (1987). *How to get your kids to eat . . . but not too much: From birth to adolescence.* Boulder, CO: Bull.

Shor, I. (1992). *Empowering education: Critical thinking for social change.* Chicago: The University of Chicago Press.

Shulman, L.S. (1986). Those who understand: Knowledge growth in teaching. *Educational Researcher, 15*(2), 4-14.

Shulman, L.S. (1987). Knowledge and teaching: Foundations of the new reform. *Harvard Educational Review, 57*(1), 1-22.

Silver, H.F., Strong, R.W., & Perini, M.J. (2000). *So each may learn: Integrating learning styles and multiple intelligences.* Alexandria, VA: Association for Supervision and Curriculum Development.

Simmons, D.C., Gunn, B., Smith, S.B., & Kameenui, E.J. (1994). Phonological awareness: Applications of instructional design. *Learning Disabilities Forum, 19,* 7-10.

Slafer, A., & Cahill, K. (1995). *Why design? Activities and projects from the national building museum.* Chicago: Chicago Review Press.

Spady, W.G. (1994). Choosing outcomes of significance. *Educational Leadership, 51*(6), 18-22.

Stanley, D. (2000). *Michelangelo.* New York: HarperCollins.

Stoy, D. (2000). Developing intercultural competence: An action plan for health educators. *Journal of Health Education, 31*(1), 16-19, 36.

Strickland, D., & Schickedanz, J. (2004). *Learning about print in preschool: Working with letters, words, and beginning links with phoneme awareness.* Newark, DE: International Reading Association.

Strong, R.W., Silver, H.F., & Perini, M.J. (2001). *Teaching what matters most: Standards and strategies for raising student achievement.* Alexandria, VA: Association for Supervision and Curriculum Development.

Tileston, D.W. (2004). *What every teacher should know about learning, memory, and the brain.* Thousand Oaks, CA: Corwin Press.

Treichel, M. (2006). Interfaith Center for Peace, Columbus, OH. Adapted and expanded from materials created for the National Dialogues on Anti-Racism, Episcopal Church in the USA, 2nd ed., 1999.

Tyler, R.W. (1949). *Basic principles of curriculum and instruction.* Chicago: University of Chicago Press.

U.S. Centers for Disease Control and Prevention. (2007a). Coordinated school health program model. Retrieved from www.cdc.gov/Healthy Youth/CSHP.

U.S. Centers for Disease Control and Prevention. (2007b). Health protection goals fact sheet: Goals for the 21st century. Retrieved from www.cdc.gov/about/goals. htm.

U.S. Department of Health and Human Services. (2000). *Healthy People 2010*. Washington, DC: Author.

Ubbes, V.A. (1999, Winter). Advocacy and teaming on behalf of adolescents: Who are they and what do they need? *HIV Prevention & Comprehensive School Health Education Project Newsletter, 5*(1), 4-6. Reston, VA: American Association for Health Education.

Ubbes, V.A. (2004). *Multiple intelligences: Different ways to educate for health.* Mason, OH: Thomson Learning.

Ubbes, V.A., & Ward, R.M. (2007). Design of a conceptual model for the study of education, health, and communication: Professional preparation issues. *Californian Journal of Health Promotion, 5*(1), 30-38. Retrieved from www. csuchico.edu/cjhp/5/1/030-038-ubbes.pdf

Ubbes, V.A., Black, J.M., & Ausherman, J.A. (1999). Constructing knowledge for understanding in health education: The role of critical and creative thinking skills within constructivism theory. *Journal of Health Education, 30*(1), 32-38.

Ubbes, V.A., Cottrell, R.R., Ausherman, J.J., Black, J.M., Wilson, P., & Gill, C. (1999). Professional preparation of elementary teachers in Ohio: Status of K-6 health education. *Journal of School Health, 69*(1), 29-32.

Ubbes, V.A., Hall, T.L., & Falk, C.A. (2004). *Modules for teaching and learning about health education: A study of guiding questions, essential readings, critical concepts, and mental models* (2nd ed.). Mason, OH: Thomson.

Van Hoose, J., Strahan, D., & L'Esperance, M. (2001). *Promoting harmony: Young adolescent development and school practices.* Westerville, OH: National Middle School Association.

Veal, W.R., and MaKinster, J.G. (1999). Pedagogical content knowledge taxonomies. *Electronic Journal of Science Education, 3*(4). http://wolfweb.unr. edu/homepage/crowther/ejse/vealmak.html.

Verdich, E. (2003). *Teeth are not for biting.* Minneapolis: Free Spirit.

Verdich, E. (2004). *Feet are not for kicking.* Minneapolis: Free Spirit.

Vygotsky, L.S. (1962). *Thought and language.* Cambridge, MA: MIT Press.

Vygotsky, L.S. (1978). *Mind in society* (M. Cole, Trans.). Cambridge, MA: Harvard University Press.

Wallbank, W., Taylor, A.M., & Bailkey, N.M. (1975). *Civilization past and present* (4th ed). Glenview, IL: Scott, Foresman and Company.

Walton, J., Hoerr, S., Heine, L., Frost, S., Roisen, D., & Berkimer, M. (1999). Physical activity and states of change in fifth and sixth graders. *Journal of School Health, 69*(7): 285-289.

Wheeler, Terrence. (1995). *Name, claim, reframe, tame, aim, don't blame.* Columbus, OH: Ohio Commission on Dispute Resolution and Conflict Management.

Wheeler, Terrence. (2004). *Choosing a conflict management style.* Columbus, OH: Ohio Commission on Dispute Resolution and Conflict Management.

Williams, R.C. (2003). *The historian's toolbox: A student's guide to the theory and craft of history.* Armonk, NY: M.E. Sharpe.

Willis, J. (2006). *Research-based strategies to ignite student learning: Insights from a neurologist and classroom teacher.* Alexandria, VA: Association for Supervision and Curriculum Development.

Wilson, J.F. (2003). The critical link between literacy and health. *Annals of Internal Medicine, 139*(10), 875-878.

Wood, D. (2002). *A quiet place.* New York: Simon & Schuster.

Wooley, S. (1995). Behavior mapping: A tool for identifying priorities for health education curricula and instruction. *Journal of Health Education, 26*(4), 202.

Wright, S.P., Horn, S.P., & Sanders, W.L. (1997). Teacher and classroom context effects on student achievement: Implications for teacher evaluation. *Journal of Personnel Evaluation in Education, 11*: 57-67.

Wurman, R.S. (1989). *Information anxiety.* New York: Doubleday.

Young, E. (1992). *Seven blind mice.* New York: Scholastic.

Zobel-Nolan, A. (2005). *What I like about me! A book celebrating differences.* Pleasantville, NY: Reader's Digest Children's Publishing.

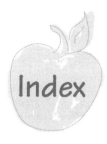

Index

*Note:* The italicized *f* and *t* following page numbers refer to figures and tables, respectively.

**A**
abstract questioning cues 55
access, concept of 28-29
Ackerman, D. 199
action plans 112, 113
action potentials 111
adolescence 65
aesthetics 13, 17*f*, 152
Agassi, M. 93
aggressive communication style 70-71*t*
Ajzen, Icek 85
Allegrante, J.P. x, 32
Angelo, T.A. 61
ANTS *vs.* bugs 208-209*t*
apple, as wellness metaphor 38-39, 40
appointment with colleague exercise 179, 180
Aristotle 76
Armstrong, T. 80, 81, 96
assertive communication style 70-71*t*
assessments 61
Ausherman, J. xii, 58-59, 132, 212
automatic negative thinking 69*t*
avoidance level of relating 204*f*

**B**
Bailkey, N.M. 76
*Basic Principles of Curriculum and Instruction* (Tyler) 147
behaviorism 53, 55
Benhar, M. 100
Bennett, Jon 44-45
Berk, R.A. 107
Berman, M. 57
Bibeau, D. 34
Binet, Alfred 100
Bjornstad, E.K. 32-33
Black, J.M. xii, 58-59, 132
Blumenfeld-Jones, D. 152
Blythe, T. 50, 101

Bobbitt, Franklin 147
bodily kinesthetic intelligence 97*t*, 99*t*, 101, 104, 140*t*
body-brain compatibility 71-73
Bonaguro, J.A. 73, 115
books, for living and learning
    *Double-Dip Feelings* (Cain) 209
    *Hands Are Not for Hitting* (Agassi) 93
    *Hands* (Ehlert) 92-93
    *Is There Really a Human Race?* (Curtis and Cornell) 46-47
    *Made by Hand* (Goldish) 93
    *The Three Questions* (Muth) 20
    *Tools* (Morris and Heyman) 175
    *26 Big Things Small Hands Do* (Paratore) 93
    *What I Like About Me!* (Zobel-Nolan) 160
    *When Cody Became a Mouse Potato* (Nygard and Koonce) 126
    *Words Are Not for Hurting* (Agassi) 93
Boyer, Ernest 17
Bredeson, P.V. 57-58, 164
Briggs Myers, Isabel 176
Brooks, J.G. 52, 150
Brooks, M.G. 52
Brown, D. 57
bugs *vs.* ANTS 208-209*t*
Bunting, C.E. 64-65

**C**
Cahill, K. 57
Cain, Barbara 209
Calvin, John 76
*The Canterbury Tales* (Chaucer) 76
cardiovascular system, river metaphor 197
caring level of relating 204*f*
Carpenter, B.S. 148-149
CDC. *See* U.S. Centers for Disease Control and Prevention
change 13, 17-19, 61, 189

change orders 59-60, 60-62
Chapman, C. 27
Chaucer, Geoffrey 76
children
 access to curriculum 26
 children's literature 129-130
 communication with body gestures 87
 giving space to 41
 in instructional groupings 82
 interaction with 24-26
 learning how to observe 30-31
 learning listening skills 102-103
 living through major disasters 7, 67-68
 observing as human beings 23-24
 patterns of action 25
 understanding function of print 82
Children's Picture Book Database xi, 20, 209
Clandinin, D.J. x, 58
co-curriculum 202
cognition 35, 144
cognitive-behavioral responses 10
cognitive-emotional bugs 70t
collaborative teaching-learning 114
colleagues, listening to 30
Columbus, Christopher 79
comfort zone, moving in and out of 196, 197
common interests level of relating 204f
communication
 complexity of process 88
 continuum of closed to open 193-194
 health communication 106-107
 information signals for 140t
 interpersonal communication 87
 knowing multiple ways of 105
 levels of relating 204f
 media and formats 97t
 school standards for 87
 skills for conflict management 12, 13
 teachers' awareness of different forms 98
communication styles 70-71t
community factors, ecological model 32
community of truth 36-37
compare and contrast 167, 176-177, 178, 182, 185
Concept-Based Curriculum and Instruction (Erickson) 108
conceptual design 108, 109t
conflict, relationship with stress 4f
conflict management 11f, 12, 13, 14-16f
Connelly, F.M. x, 58
Connor, M. 85
Constructing the Knowledges (Dobrin) 130-131
Constructivist Pre-Lesson Template 153-154f

constructivist theory
 about 51-55
 and design process 60
 in education 56
 epistemology of 163-164
 as framework for health education x, 50
 objective knowing and subjective knowing 83-85
 zone of proximal development 85-86
contextual knowledge 111, 164
contextual model of human expertise 141, 142f, 143-144
convergent thinking 110
cooperative conflict-response styles 11f
cooperative learning 56, 162, 167, 179, 180
cooperative problem solving 14f
Cornell, Laura 46-47
Costa, A.L. 54, 55
Cottrell, R.R. 212
Creativity in Education and Learning (Cropley) 110
Cropley, A.J. 110, 111
Cross, K.P. 61
cultural identity 5f
cultural sensitivity 68-69
culture, epitome of 6-7
curriculum
 aesthetics and curriculum thinking 152
 children's access to 26
 co-curriculum 202
 historical and philosophical perspectives 147-149
 preK-12 health curriculum problems 116-117
 review not equitable for health education 117
 synergy with pedagogy 148
 as text 145-147
The Curriculum (Bobbitt) 147
curriculum coordinators 119-120
Curtis, Jamie Lee 46-47

**D**
Danielson, C. 51
Dante Alighieri 76
Darling-Hammond, L. 163
debate 182, 194
declarative knowledge 57, 111, 164-165
Deline, J. 63
Derryberry, Matthew x
design
 about 56-57
 architectural metaphor 58-59
 of body 23-24
 elements of 13, 17f
 environment's role in 62-63
 as inquiry-based approach 110

as inquiry process 57-58
and style 81-82
developmental appropriateness 64-68
Dewey, J. 51, 147
dialogue 182, 194
DiClemente, C.C. 85
didactic discourse 194*t*
differentiated instruction 26
disasters 6, 7, 68
discipline 194*t*
discussion 182, 194
divergent thinking 110
Dobrin, S.I. 130-131
domain-specific information 102
Donahue, R.E. 32-33
double-dip feelings 201
Dreifus, C. 75
dysfunctional thinking 69

**E**
ecological model 32-34, 33*f*, 138-141
Eddy, J.M. 32-33, 34
educating for health. *See also* health education
and change orders 60-62
constructivist approaches 55
in faith-based institutions 78
language and literacy roles 103-104
literacy in 82-83
need for skill development 11, 13
in other places 32
philosophy for 80-81, 134-135
with positive disposition 67
problem solving in 110-111
professional skills used for 146*f*
as synonym for health education x
theoretical mapping of three learning zones 172
education
attendance patterns 5-6
bias in 137
bridges into health ix-x
broken paradoxes of 7
constructivism in 56
interaction with health professionals 56
professional teaming in education and health 119-121
structural elements of 145*f*
educator, origin of term 42
Ehlert, Lois 92-93
Eisley, Loren 68
Eisner, Elliot 31, 147
Ellison, L. 197
emotional hijacking 72
Enlightenment period 76
environment, role in design 62-63
environmental print 105-106

Enz, B.J. 105
Erickson, Lynn 108
Ericsson, A. 102
Erikson, E. 107
evidence-based instructional strategies
categories of 166*t*
design questions for 170-171*f*
examples 176-185
in health education 84-85, 165-168
improving student achievement 172
nonlinguistic representations of 170-171*f*
and patterns in pedagogy 163
as tools and patterns for all disciplines 168-169
experience, narratives of 29-30
expert performance 102
*The Exquisite Risk* (Nepo) ix, 1, 21, 49, 127, 161, 187, 211

**F**
Fahlberg, L.A. 52
Fahlberg, L.L. 52
faith, and moments of reflection 5
Falk, C.A. 38
fantasy 107-108
Faundez, A. 53
federal government 212. *See also* U.S. Centers for Disease Control and Prevention; U.S. Department of Education; U.S. Department of Health and Human Services
feedback, providing 183
feelings
and conflict management 12
double-dip feelings 201
facing own 201
focusing 8
loving feelings 198
supportive role in thinking 8-9
Fishbein, Martin 85
Fisher, B. 129
Flinders, D.J. 148
Friere, P. 53
function, as element of design 13, 17*f*
Futures Initiative (U.S. Centers for Disease Control and Prevention) 211

**G**
Galileo Galilei 77
Galley, Paul 21
Gardner, Howard
Ellison on 197
identity formation 6
intelligence 100, 101-102
language as play 107
mastery of discipline 50
multiple intelligences theory 33, 96, 110-111, 196

Geertz, C. 68, 128
Gerard, M.R. 105-106, 107-108
German culture 133
Gillmore, M.R. 85
Given, B.K. 86, 199
Glanz, K. 34
Goldish, M. 93
graphic organizers 167
Green, L.W. 115
Greenberg, J.S. 38, 39, 40, 190
Greenfield, G. 203
greeting level of relating 204*f*
Gregory, G. 27
Grossman, P. 164
Guilford, J.P. 110
Gunn, B. 106

**H**
habits of health 54-55, 113-116, 167, 178, 195
habits of mind 54-55, 113-116, 167, 195
Hall, E.T. 68
Hall, T.L. 38
Halpern, D.F. 52
Hanley, M.S. 128
harmony 62-63
Harwayne, S. 7
Hawkins, Jeff 95
Hawks, S.R. 198
Haynes, J. 175
health
  bridges into education ix-x
  components of 38
  concepts taught in other disciplines 117-118
  as cooperation between cells 21
  as curriculum of life 145
  foundational to learning 84
  habits of 54-55
  honoring dimensions of 24-26, 191
  and literacy 104-106
  multiple professional perspectives in 136-138
  from paradox of wellness and illness 18
  professional teaming in education and health 119-121
  promotion via practice and rehearsal 50
  quality of living related to 17
health behavior 34, 136
health communication 106-107, 136
health coordinating councils 120
health education. *See also* educating for health
  bridging educational theories into xi
  building infrastructure for 118-119
  changing disciplinary perspectives 137
  cognitive perspective of 132

evidence-based instructional strategies 84-85, 165-168
  as lifelong connected experience 134
  mapping educational theories into 132
  objectives of *Educating for Health* xii-xiii
  performance standards 150
  planned and incidental learning episodes 114
  professional stories of 131
  studies of Ubbes 133
  theoretical frameworks ix-x
health education perspectives 136
health enhancement 73-74
healthful practices 113-116
health literacy 105
health professionals, meeting with teachers 212-213
health promoter, thinking as 74-75
health-related skills, assessing 183
health science perspectives 136
*Healthy People 2010* (U.S. Department of Health and Human Services) 68
heart, as symbol of love 198
Heyman, K. 175
hierarchies 42
Hillman, S.B. 65
hooks, bell 80-81
Horn, S.P. 163
Hull, M.L. 198
human beings
  as human doings 144
  observing children as 23-24
  reflection on role as 23
  as self-smart and people smart 107
human body 65, 134-135, 190
human interactions, importance of 200
human language, emergence of 75
human senses
  acknowledging role of 190
  attention to environmental cues 135
  in ecological model 138-141
  in information processing 102-103
  star symbol 39, 40*f*
human well-being model 41
Hyerle, D. 169, 170*f*

**I**
identity formation 4, 5-6, 18, 139*f*
information
  as in formation 35, 77
  holistic approach to 9
  integrating with prior knowledge 195
  sharing between teachers and students 202
  signals used for communication 140*t*
informational texts 129-130
information overload 66-67

information processing 106
inquiry 53, 54*t*
inquiry-based approach x, 52
institutional factors, ecological model 32
intelligence, defined 100-102
International Society for Technology in Education xi
Internet. *See* Web links
interpersonal communication 87
interpersonal factors, ecological model 32
interpersonal intelligence 197
interpersonal learners 27, 28*t*, 34, 139*f*, 176-177
interpersonal social intelligence 101
interpretations, based on what is not 86-87
intimacy level of relating 204*f*
intrapersonal factors, ecological model 32
intrapersonal intelligence 197
intrapersonal introspective intelligence 101
Irwin, R.L. 128
*Is There Really a Human Race?* (Curtis and Cornell) 46-47

**J**
Janesick, V.J. 149
judgment, of self and others 68-69
Jung, Carl x, 176

**K**
Kallick, B. 54
Kameenui, E.J. 106
Kasprzyk, D. 85
Kepler, Johannes 77
King, A. 53
King, P.M. 51
knowledge
contextual knowledge 111, 164
declarative knowledge 57, 111, 164-165
historical significance of knowledge construction 75-78
multiple sources of 143*t*
pedagogical content knowledge 164-165
pedagogical knowledge 164
personal practical knowledge 31
procedural knowledge 57, 111, 165
sources of 141-144
structure of 112*t*
subject matter knowledge 164
when ruled by church 75-78
*Knowledge as Design* (Perkins) 169, 171
knowledge gap 36
knowledge structures 50. *See also* constructivist theory
Koonce, S. 126
Kornhaber, M. 33
Kreuter, M.W. 85, 115

**L**
Langston, L.P. 148-149
language
advancing study of health education 189
elements of 99*t*
emergence of human language 75
as play 107-108
role in educating for health 103-104
signs and symbols for 96-98
structure, function, and aesthetic forms 98, 100
Lasher, W. 46
Latin, in Middle Ages 76
Lazear, D. 33-34, 107
Leamnson, R. 166
learners
attending to role of human senses 135
constructing information to learn 52
focus on 31
as lesson co-designers 66
subject matter interaction 53
teacher interaction 42-43
learning
body-brain compatibility 71-73
cooperative learning 56, 162, 167, 179, 180
cultural sensitivity 68-69
developmental appropriateness 64-68
establishing conditions for 64
health enhancement 73-74
mystery of life and learning 8-9
objective *vs.* subjective structures 35-37
safe and supportive environment for 205-207
sensory patterns 57
service learning 56
tailoring to individual 9
learning environment, establishing 63
learning styles
about 26-27
example of compare and contrast strategy 176-177
interpersonal learners 27, 28*t*, 34, 139*f*, 176-177
mastery learners 27, 28*t*, 139*f*, 176
patterns of similarities and differences 28-29
self-expressive learners 27, 28*t*, 139*f*, 177
understanding learners 27, 28*t*, 139*f*, 177
ways to access information 141
learning styles theory x, 172
L'Esperance, M. 108
Lesson Implementation Plan 156*f*
Lesson Implementation Schedule 157*f*
Lesson Preplanning Outline 155*f*
lessons 25, 59-60, 66, 196
Lester, Julius 80

*Let's Talk About Race* (Lester) 80
life
  dealing with changes 3-4
  establishing quality of 7-8
  health as curriculum of 145
  as journey into core of identity 22
  mystery of life and learning 8-9
"listening" skill 184
literacy 82-83, 103-104, 104-106, 129
literature, children's 129-130
logical mathematical intelligence 99*t*, 101, 140*t*
loving feelings 198
Lowery, L. 55
Luther, Martin 77

**M**
Maglich, Hope 123
Magolda, M.B. 51
make-believe 108
MaKinster, J.G. 164
Malow-Iroff, M. 100
Martin, S. 100
Marzano, Robert J. 164, 165, 168, 170*f*, 174
mastery learners 27, 28*t*, 139*f*, 176
McDermott, M. 148
McLeroy, K.R. 34
McMillan, B. 85
media messages 116
Medvic, E.F. 129
Merton, T. 7
metaphors, as instructional strategy 57-58
Michelangelo 78
Middle Ages 75-76
Milbratz, Abby 158-159
Montano, D.E. 85
Moran, S. 33
Morris, A. 175
Mullen, C.A. 147
multiple intelligences theory
  about 33-34
  communication 97*t*, 107
  components of 101, 103
  in education x, 172
  language elements 99*t*
  in problem solving 110-111
  relationships 196
  sources of 96
*Multiple Intelligences* (Ubbes) 191
musical rhythmical intelligence 97*t*, 99*t*, 101, 140*t*
Muth, Jon 20

**N**
National Health Education Standards 52, 63, 116, 134, 149-150, 151, 160, 172
National Research Council 108
naturalist environmental intelligence 99*t*, 101, 140*t*

Nepo, Mark
  *The Exquisite Risk* ix, 1, 21, 49, 127, 161, 187, 211
  life changes 3-4, 159-160
  on relationships 206
  science and conscience 92
  spaces in between 124
  web of life 174
  wellness 45
networks 42
Newell, A. 102
nonlinguistic representations 182, 183
Nummedal, S.G. 52
Nygard, B. 126

**O**
Oberman, L.M. 135
objective inquiry 185
objectives, setting 183
objectivism 83-85
objectivist myth of knowing 36-37
*On Intelligence* (Hawkins and Blakeslee) 95
ontology 22
Owen, N. 32

**P**
pace 25-26, 63
Palmer, P.J. 3, 4, 7, 8, 37, 45, 83-84, 159
Paratore, C. 93
passive communication style 70-71*t*
patterns, observing 162-163
Paul, Richard 84
pedagogical content knowledge 164-165
pedagogical knowledge 164
pedagogy 64, 148, 163-164, 203
peer education 162
performances of understanding 50
Perini, M.J. 27, 28, 34, 176
Perkins, David 50, 169, 171
personal identity 4, 5*f*
personal practical knowledge 31
personal skills 178
personal well-being, fostering culture of 9-10
phonemic awareness 82, 106
Piaget, J. x, 39, 51
Pinar, W.F. 147
place, contextual issues of 196-197
Planned Behavior, Theory of 85
Plato 76
play 107-108
Postman, N. 137
power 83, 146
PRE-vention work 115-116
preventive medicine 73
Prior, J.O. 105-106, 107-108
private identity 4, 5*f*
procedural knowledge 57, 111, 165

Prochaska, J.O.  85
professional practices  146*f*, 202-203
professional preparation standards  151*t*
Protestantism  77
puberty  65
public identity  4, 5*f*
public policies, and ecological model  32

**Q**
quality issues  149-151
question probes  185
*A Quiet Place* (Wood)  195
quiet time  194-195
quilts, as metaphors  128

**R**
race, concept of  80-81
Ramachandran, V.S.  135
reflection
   individual differences regarding  196
   on personal and professional life  181
   plans for reflective practice  193-195
   on teaching practices  31
reflex system  72
Reformation  77
relational pedagogy  203
relationships
   as connecting macroconcept  190
   explained  196
   at heart of instructional design  202
   importance of  199-202
   Nepo on  206
   with people  191-193
   working at  203, 205
Renaissance  75-76, 78
Reynolds, W.M.  147
Richins, P.M.  198
river, as cardiovascular system metaphor
   197
role models  31, 50

**S**
Sallis, J.F.  32
Sanchez, R.  130
Sanders, W.L.  163
scaffolding process  82
Schickedanz, J.  82-83
schools, mission and vision statements  30
Schutte, Carolyn Stewart  207-208
self, acceptance of  206
self-authorship  51
self-discovery  2-3
self-expressive learners  27, 28*t*, 139*f*, 177
self identity  5*f*
semantics, defined  98
semiotics  98, 104
sensory information  71-73
sensory-motor responses  10, 72

sensory-motor skills  144
separate interests level of relating  204*f*
September 11 disaster  6, 7
service learning  56
*Seven Blind Mice* (Young)  22
sharing level of relating  204*f*
Shor, I.  53
Shulman, L.S.  164
Silver, H.F.  27, 28, 34, 176
Simmons, D.C.  106
Simon, H.A.  102
Simon, Theodore  100
skill development  11, 13, 149, 150*f*
*Skin Again* (hooks)  80-81
Slafer, A.  57
Slattery, P.  147
Sleet, D.A.  x, 32
Smith, S.B.  106
smoking-cessation programs  34
social interaction level of relating  204*f*
social skills  178
social web of meaning  128
society, integrating self with  82
Socrates  76
sound mind, in sound body  133
space, contextual issues of  196-197
speech, as conflict in personal relationships
   87
spiritual health  198
Stanford-Binet Intelligence Scale  100
Stanley, D.  78, 79
star, as symbol  27, 38-39, 138, 141
Steckler, A.  34
stories, ways to structure  128-129
Stoy, D.  68
Strahan, D.  108
stress  4*f*, 7-8, 72
Strickland, D.  82-83
Strong, R.W.  27, 28, 34, 176
structure, as element of design  13, 17*f*
student-centered instruction  61-62
students. *See* learners
subjective inquiry  185
subjectivism  83-85
subject matter knowledge  164
summarizing  183
sunlight metaphor  67
Sykes, G.  163
symbol systems  96

**T**
Taubman, P.M.  147
Taylor, A.M.  76
teachers
   as changing learners and leaders  3-4
   education of  212
   interaction with students  42-43
   as interpreters of patterns  162-163

teachers *(continued)*
   meeting with health professionals 212-213
   provocative materials used by 192-193
   sending vibrations 192
   sensitivity toward body language 193
   tree metaphor 29-30
teacher voices
   Abby Milbratz 158-159
   Carolyn Stewart Schutte 207-208
   Hope Maglich 123
   Jennifer Lane 173-174
   Jon Bennett 44-45
   Valerie A. Ubbes 18-19, 89-91, 173-174
teaching
   environmental and cultural contexts 43
   heart and soul of 198
   objective *vs.* subjective structures 35-37
Thalman, R.L. 198
theory, compared to story 130-131
Theory of Reasoned Action 85
thoughts, focusing 8
three-part thinking model 84
touch 199
transdisciplinary concepts 109*t*
transformative thinking 148
Transtheoretical Model of Behavior Change 85
Turner Club 133, 134
Tyler, Ralph 147

**U**
Ubbes, V.A.
   Constructing Knowledge for Understanding in Health Education xii, 58-59, 65, 132
   Design of a Conceptual Model for the Study of Education 97
   *Modules for Teaching and Learning* 38
   *Multiple Intelligences* 34, 45-46, 191
   personal philosophy of 133-134
   philosophy of learning and teaching 18-19
   planning for daily instruction 89-91
   professional philosophy of 132
   Professional Preparation of Elementary Teachers in Ohio 212
uncooperative conflict-response styles 11*f*
understanding learners 27, 28*t*, 139*f*, 177
U.S. Centers for Disease Control and Prevention 120, 211-212
U.S. Department of Education 212
U.S. Department of Health and Human Services 212

**V**
Van Hoose, J. 108
Veal, W.R. 164
verbal linguistic intelligence 97*t*, 99*t*, 101, 103, 140*t*
visual spatial intelligence 97*t*, 99*t*, 101, 140*t*
Vygtosky, Lev x, 51, 85-86, 107

**W**
Wallbank, W. 76
Walton, J. 85
Ward, R.M. 97
ways to be 24-26
Web links
   Children's Picture Book Database xi, 20, 209
   communication channels used 126
   educational formats used 126
   evidence-based instructional strategies 174-175
   human senses subtext 125*f*
   language elements subtext 126
   National Health Education Standards 160
   public health campaigns 124-125*t*
   VARK sensory learning 92
   wellness policy in American schools 46
Webster, R.D. 32-33
wellness 9-10, 38-41, 65
"Wellness Perspectives for Adolescents" 40
"when someone bothers you" skill 183
*Why Design?* (Slafer and Cahill) 57
Williams, R.C. 75
Willis, J. xii
Wood, Douglas 195
Wooley, S. 115
world-centric view 52
World Health Organization 105
World Wide Web. *See* web links
Wray, R.J. 85
Wright, S.P. 163
Wurman, R.S. 52
Wycliff, John 76

**Y**
"The Year of the Healthy Child" 211
YMCA, influence of 134
Young, Ed 22

**Z**
Zobel-Nolan, A. 160
zone of proximal development 85-86
Zwingli, Ulrich 76

# About the Author

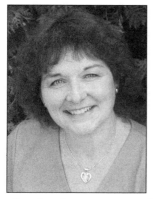

**Valerie A. Ubbes, PhD, CHES,** is an associate professor in kinesiology and health at Miami University. She has taught pedagogy courses since 1980 and has developed three pedagogy courses for which she has published three books.

Dr. Ubbes is also project director of the Children's Picture Book Database at Miami University (www.lib.muohio.edu/pictbks). Her multidisciplinary database was recognized by the International Society for Technology in Education (2005) as one of the 101 best Web sites for elementary teachers. In 1995, she wrote the first integrated curriculum book that was aligned with the National Health Education Standards, and she has served as the health in education network facilitator for the Association for Supervision and Curriculum Development. She is an active member of the American Association for Health Education.

In her spare time, Dr. Ubbes enjoys landscaping, flower gardening, bicycling, reading, playing her bassoon, and traveling with her family. Her life goal is to promote human well-being across the life span, leading to a higher quality of life and learning for all.